Medical Radiology

Diagnostic Imaging

The book series *Medical Radiology – Diagnostic Imaging* provides accurate and up-to-date overviews about the latest advances in the rapidly evolving field of diagnostic imaging and interventional radiology. Each volume is conceived as a practical and clinically useful reference book and is developed under the direction of an experienced editor, who is a world-renowned specialist in the field. Book chapters are written by expert authors in the field and are richly illustrated with high quality figures, tables and graphs. Editors and authors are committed to provide detailed and coherent information in a readily accessible and easy-to-understand format, directly applicable to daily practice.

Medical Radiology – Diagnostic Imaging covers all organ systems and addresses all modern imaging techniques and image-guided treatment modalities, as well as hot topics in management, workflow, and quality and safety issues in radiology and imaging. The judicious choice of relevant topics, the careful selection of expert editors and authors, and the emphasis on providing practically useful information, contribute to the wide appeal and ongoing success of the series. The series is indexed in Scopus.

Kanaka Durga Prasad Bhamidipaty
Rajesh Botchu
Veenadhari Bhamidipaty
Editors

Injuries in Musicians - Imaging and Management

Springer

Editors
Kanaka Durga Prasad Bhamidipaty
Department of Radiology
NRIIMS
Visakhapatnam, Andhra Pradesh, India

Veenadhari Bhamidipaty
Department of Computer Science and Engineering
GITAM University
Visakhapatnam, Andhra Pradesh, India

Rajesh Botchu
Department of Musculoskeletal Radiology
Royal Orthopaedic Hospital
Birmingham, UK

ISSN 0942-5373 ISSN 2197-4187 (electronic)
Medical Radiology
ISSN 2731-4677 ISSN 2731-4685 (electronic)
Diagnostic Imaging
ISBN 978-3-032-14364-8 ISBN 978-3-032-14365-5 (eBook)
https://doi.org/10.1007/978-3-032-14365-5

This Springer imprint is published by the registered company Springer Nature Switzerland AG
The registered company address is: Gewerbestrasse 11, 6330 Cham, Switzerland

Preface

Musicians, like athletes, are prone to a unique set of injuries resulting from repetitive movements, sustained postures, and performance-related stress. Injuries in Musicians: Imaging and Management addresses this important yet often overlooked aspect of clinical practice. As interest grows in the intersection of performing arts and medicine, this book serves as a timely and focused resource for physicians, radiologists, and rehabilitation specialists involved in the care of performing artists.

This volume provides a systematic approach to understanding music-related injuries through the combined lens of clinical expertise and imaging interpretation. The initial chapters explore the cultural and historical context of global music, classification of musical instruments, and the specific injuries associated with both vocal and instrumental performance, supported by discussions on pathophysiology and relevant radiological features.

The later sections delve into postural abnormalities, ergonomic challenges unique to musicians, and an orthopedic perspective on musculoskeletal conditions in this population. Emphasis is also placed on rehabilitation strategies, and the final chapter reflects on musical aesthetics—recognizing that full recovery encompasses not only physical function but also the restoration of artistic expression.

The editors gratefully acknowledge the valuable contributions of professionals from diverse fields. This book aims to serve as a comprehensive guide to the understanding, diagnosis, and management of music-related injuries by integrating the science of imaging with the art of medicine, ultimately supporting the health and longevity of musicians worldwide.

Visakhapatnam, Andhra Pradesh, India — Kanaka Durga Prasad Bhamidipaty
Birmingham, UK — Rajesh Botchu
Visakhapatnam, Andhra Pradesh, India — Veenadhari Bhamidipaty

Acknowledgements

Music sharpens our senses, allowing us to perceive the finest nuances in melody and harmony; similarly, radiologists identify subtle, often elusive details within medical images. This book brings these two worlds together, shedding light on the wide range of injuries that can affect musicians.

The completion of this work was made possible through the commitment and expertise of the editors, Prof. Kanaka Durga Prasad Bhamidipaty, Veenadhari Bhamidipaty, and Prof. Rajesh Botchu. Their guidance, supported by the dedication of many others, transformed this concept into reality, and I extend my heartfelt gratitude to everyone involved.

I wish to sincerely thank the doctors, allied health professionals, physiotherapists, researchers, and musicians whose work is devoted to understanding, preventing, and managing injuries related to music performance.

I am deeply appreciative of my family and friends for their constant encouragement, support, and patience during the countless hours devoted to writing and editing this manuscript.

Finally, I extend special thanks to all contributors, as well as to Springer (our publisher), Prakash Balasubramanian, and Nathalie Lhorset-Poulain, whose efforts ensured that this book was completed on time.

Contents

Introduction to Musculoskeletal and Vocal Injuries in Musicians

Durgananda Lahari Bhamidipaty,
Veenadhari Bhamidipaty, Ramarao Malla,
and Kanaka Durga Prasad Bhamidipaty

Contents

D. L. Bhamidipaty
Department of Industrial Biotechnology, Manipal Institute of Technology, Manipal, India

V. Bhamidipaty
Department of CSE, GITAM, Visakhapatnam, India

R. Malla
Department of Life Sciences, GITAM, Visakhapatnam, India

K. D. P. Bhamidipaty (✉)
Department of Radiodiagnosis, NRIIMS, Visakhapatnam, India

Abstract

Professional musicians and vocalists, akin to athletes, face significant risks of musculoskeletal and vocal injuries due to repetitive movements, awkward postures, and intense vocal exertion inherent to their craft. These performance-related injuries, including tendonitis, nerve compression syndromes, and vocal fold nodules, affect 26%–93% of instrumentalists and 11%–59% of singers, with prevalence varying due to inconsistent diagnostic criteria across studies. Diagnostic imaging, such as MRI, ultrasound, X-ray, and laryngoscopy, is critical for accurate diagnosis, with MRI detecting soft tissue pathology in over 70% of cases among string players and vocalists with persistent symptoms. This chapter introduces the epidemiology, diagnosis, and management of these injuries, emphasizing interdisciplinary approaches that integrate medical, rehabilitative, and preventive strategies to enhance performers' health, optimize functional outcomes, and sustain career longevity.

1 Introduction

The artistry of musical performance, encompassing instrumental mastery and vocal expression, demands exceptional physical and technical precision. This intensity places performers at risk for

Med Radiol Diagn Imaging (2025)

https://doi.org/10.1007/174_2025_625,
Published Online: 25 September 2025

occupational injuries that can compromise their health and professional sustainability. Playing-related musculoskeletal disorders (PRMDs) and vocal fold pathologies, such as tendonitis, carpal tunnel syndrome, vocal nodules, and muscle tension dysphonia, are prevalent yet often underdiagnosed due to limited clinician awareness and performers' reluctance to report symptoms amid competitive pressures (Kok et al. 2016; Pestana et al. 2017). These conditions arise from repetitive strain, suboptimal ergonomics, inadequate preparation, and psychosocial stressors, such as performance anxiety, which amplify physical demands. Left unaddressed, these injuries can progress to chronic pain or functional limitations, threatening performers' careers and well-being.

This book, *Injuries in Musicians: Imaging and Management*, provides clinicians, therapists, educators, and performers with a practical, evidence-based guide to address these challenges. This introductory chapter outlines the prevalence and nature of musculoskeletal and vocal injuries, highlights the critical role of imaging modalities, and introduces interdisciplinary strategies for rehabilitation and prevention. Subsequent chapters will explore specific injury patterns, advanced diagnostic techniques, and tailored interventions to support the performing arts community.

2 Scope of Injuries in Performers

Instrumentalists and vocalists face distinct yet overlapping injury profiles, driven by the unique biomechanical demands of their craft. PRMDs affect 26%–93% of musicians, a wide range reflecting inconsistent diagnostic criteria and study methodologies (Kok et al. 2016; Baadjou et al. 2016). Common conditions include overuse-related injuries such as tendonitis, tenosynovitis, and nerve compression syndromes (e.g., carpal tunnel syndrome), as well as task-specific focal dystonia, which impairs fine motor control through involuntary muscle contractions (Altenmüller and Jabusch 2010; Konczak and Abbruzzese 2013). These injuries typically manifest as pain, stiffness, numbness, or tingling, predominantly affecting the upper limbs, neck, and back.

Injury patterns vary by instrument type. String players, such as violinists and violists, frequently experience rotator cuff strain, neck spasms, and trapezius myalgia due to prolonged static postures and repetitive bow movements (Nyman et al. 2007). Pianists are prone to De Quervain's tenosynovitis (Mangukiya et al. 2019; Robinson 2003) and carpal tunnel syndrome from repetitive finger and wrist motions. Wind instrumentalists, including flautists and clarinetists, face thumb overuse and embouchure strain due to sustained lip and facial muscle engagement (Clemente et al. 2020). Percussionists report mid- and low-back pain, shoulder impingement, and knee strain from forceful, repetitive drumming and unsupported seated postures, which demand significant core endurance (Baadjou et al. 2016).

In the Indian context, musicians playing traditional instruments like the sitar, tabla, or mridangam often perform and practice while seated cross-legged on the floor or low platforms, a posture that imposes unique biomechanical stress on the hip, knee, and ankle joints. Prolonged cross-legged sitting can lead to hip flexor tightness, knee ligament strain, and ankle instability, particularly in tabla or mridangam players who maintain this position for hours during rigorous practice sessions or performances. For sitar or veena players, the forward-leaning posture exacerbates lower back strain and may contribute to hip osteoarthritis or patellofemoral pain syndrome over time, especially if ergonomic support, such as cushions or elevated seating, is absent. These lower limb injuries, compounded by repetitive hand and finger movements, increase the risk of chronic musculoskeletal issues in Indian musicians, necessitating targeted interventions to address both upper and lower body demands.

Vocalists, affected by voice disorders in 11%–59% of cases, develop vocal fold nodules (Fig. 1) (Kelchner et al. 2003), polyps, or muscle tension dysphonia from repetitive phonation, improper breath support, or excessive vocal intensity (Pestana et al. 2017). These

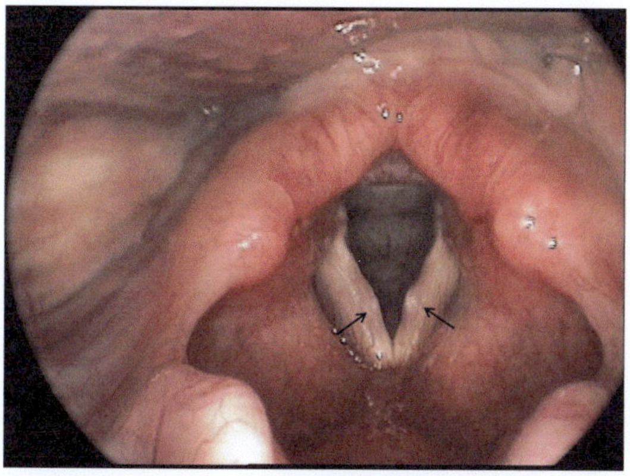

Fig. 1 Laryngoscopy showing bilateral vocal nodules (Kelchner et al. 2003)

conditions present as hoarseness, vocal fatigue, or pitch instability, often accompanied by musculoskeletal issues like cervical spine strain and temporomandibular joint (TMJ) dysfunction due to prolonged vocal effort. Indian vocalists, particularly those performing classical genres like Hindustani or Carnatic music, may also experience lower limb strain from prolonged seated postures during performances, mirroring the musculoskeletal challenges faced by instrumentalists. Risk factors across performers include prolonged practice or singing duration (often exceeding 4–6 h daily), sudden increases in performance intensity, inadequate warm-ups or cool-downs, poor ergonomic setups, and psychosocial stressors like performance anxiety or career pressures (Kaufman-Cohen and Ratzon 2011). For vocalists, additional risks include dehydration, vocal overuse during illness, and lack of vocal coaching, which exacerbate laryngeal strain. The variability in prevalence data underscores the need for standardized diagnostic frameworks to enhance recognition and facilitate early intervention.

A 28-year-old Carnatic vocalist presented with vocal fatigue during prolonged alapana sessions. Laryngoscopy revealed early vocal fold nodules (Fig. 1) (Kelchner et al. 2003), likely due to repetitive phonation without adequate breath support. Voice therapy and ergonomic posture adjustments resolved symptoms within 3 months.

3 Key Points for Clinicians

- Musculoskeletal and vocal injuries affect up to 93% of instrumentalists and 59% of vocalists, driven by repetitive strain, poor ergonomics, and psychosocial stressors.
- Early recognition through targeted clinical assessment prevents chronicity and career curtailment.
- Imaging modalities (MRI, ultrasound, X-ray, laryngoscopy) enhance diagnostic precision, guiding tailored interventions.
- Multidisciplinary care, integrating therapy, ergonomic adjustments, and psychological support, optimizes functional outcomes.

4 Role of Diagnostic Imaging

Accurate diagnosis drives effective injury management, with imaging modalities providing critical insights into underlying pathologies. X-rays assess bony structures, identifying fractures or degenerative changes, such as osteoarthritis in a guitarist's finger joints or a tabla player's knee, to rule out structural causes of pain. MRI, highly sensitive for soft tissue evaluation, detects pathology in over 70% of cases involving tendon tears, nerve compressions, disc herniations, or vocal fold lesions (Kok et al. 2016). For instance, MRI can confirm rotator cuff tendinopathy (Fig. 2) (Yubran et al. 2024) in a violinist, median nerve compression in a pianist, or hip joint effusion in a sitar player with persistent pain. In vocalists, MRI may reveal TMJ dysfunction or cervical disc issues contributing to vocal strain.

Musculoskeletal ultrasound, a dynamic and cost-effective tool, enables real-time visualization of moving structures. For example, it can assess tendon friction during simulated bowing in violinists, identifying tenosynovitis, or evaluate TMJ dynamics in vocalists with jaw pain, guiding precise corticosteroid injections. In the Indian context, ultrasound is particularly valuable for assessing knee ligament strain or ankle instability in tabla players, where dynamic imaging captures joint movement under stress. Laryngoscopy, criti-

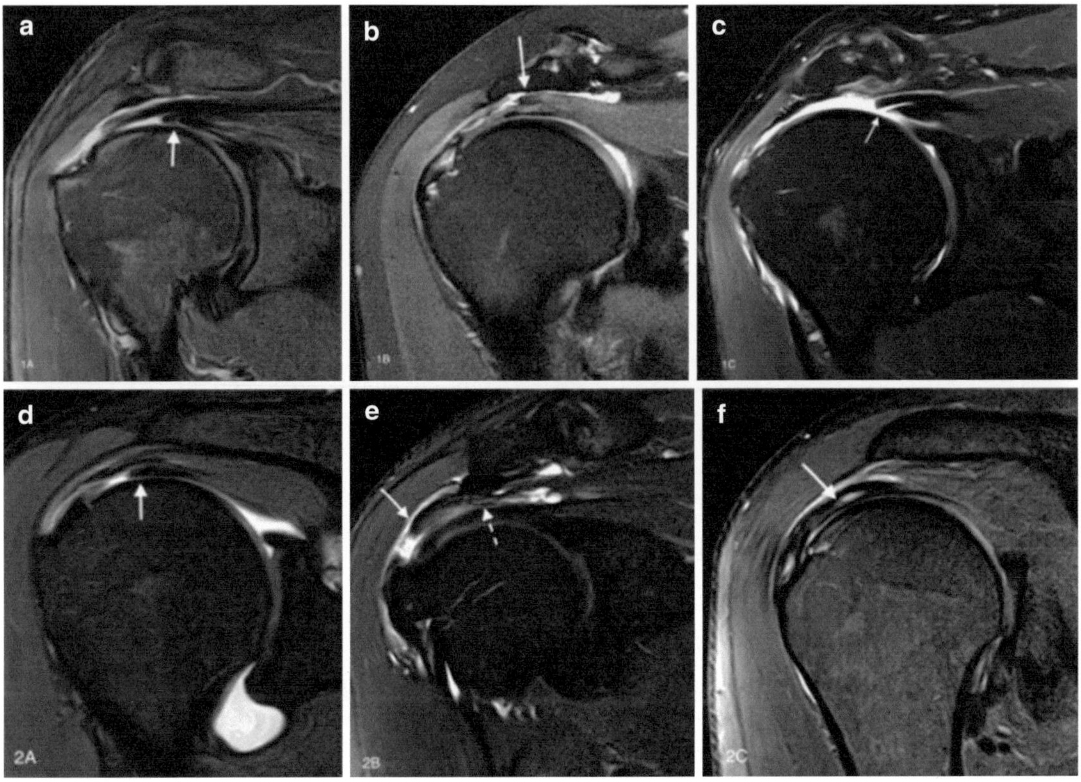

Fig. 2 An MRI scan showing rotator cuff tendinopathy, with annotations highlighting tendon thickening and inflammation relevant to violinists' shoulder strain (Yubran et al. 2024)

cal for vocalists, visualizes vocal fold pathology, detecting nodules (Fig. 1) (Kelchner et al. 2003) or polyps in up to 60% of singers with chronic hoarseness (Pestana et al. 2017). A clinical scenario illustrates this: a flautist with wrist pain may undergo ultrasound to confirm extensor tendon inflammation, followed by MRI to rule out nerve involvement. Similarly, a tabla player with knee pain may require X-ray to exclude osteoarthritis, complemented by ultrasound to assess ligament integrity. A vocalist with persistent hoarseness may undergo laryngoscopy to identify mucosal changes, with MRI to evaluate cervical contributors. A combined approach—X-ray for bony issues, ultrasound for dynamic assessment, MRI for complex soft tissue pathology, and laryngoscopy for vocal fold evaluation—ensures diagnostic precision, enabling tailored treatment plans that address the unique biomechanical demands of each performer.

5 Management and Prevention Framework

Effective management of performers' injuries requires an individualized, multidisciplinary approach addressing physical and psychosocial factors. Conservative management, the cornerstone of treatment, includes relative rest, nonsteroidal anti-inflammatory drugs (NSAIDs), and specialized physical or voice therapy tailored to performers' needs. Therapists with performing arts expertise strengthen weak muscles, stretch tight structures, and retrain techniques to restore function. For example, percussionists with low-back pain benefit from core-strengthening exercises, while pianists with tendonitis require targeted hand therapy to improve dexterity (Baadjou et al. 2016). Vocalists with nodules undergo voice therapy to optimize breath support and reduce laryngeal tension, guided by speech-language pathologists (Pestana et al. 2017).

In the Indian context, musicians seated cross-legged for extended periods benefit from targeted interventions to address hip, knee, and ankle strain. Physical therapy for tabla or sitar players includes hip flexor stretches, knee stabilization exercises, and ankle mobility drills to counteract prolonged static postures. Ergonomic interventions, such as cushioned mats or low stools to elevate seating, reduce joint compression and improve circulation in the lower limbs. For example, a tabla player with knee pain may use a supportive cushion to minimize patellofemoral stress, while a sitar player adjusts posture to reduce hip flexor tightness.

Ergonomic interventions for all performers minimize strain. For instrumentalists, optimizing chair height for percussionists, modifying bow grip for string players, or using padded key covers for pianists mitigates repetitive stress. Vocalists benefit from microphone positioning to reduce vocal effort and posture correction to minimize cervical strain. Splints or vocal rest support recovery, particularly for acute injuries. In refractory cases, corticosteroid injections (Fig. 3) (Tumpaj et al. 2022) provide targeted relief, while surgery, such as vocal fold microsurgery or carpal tunnel release, is reserved for severe cases. Multidisciplinary teams, including physicians, physical therapists, voice coaches, and psychologists, address performance anxiety to optimize outcomes.

Prevention is critical to sustaining performers' careers. Education on warm-ups, stretching, and gradual increases in practice or singing volume conditions the body and voice, reducing injury risk. For instrumentalists, warm-up routines targeting specific muscle groups (e.g., shoulder stretches for violinists, hip and knee mobility exercises for tabla players) enhance resilience, while vocalists benefit from vocal warm-ups and hydration protocols to maintain laryngeal health (Baadjou et al. 2016; Pestana et al. 2017). In the Indian context, musicians incorporate dynamic stretches before and after practice to maintain hip, knee, and ankle flexibility, reducing joint

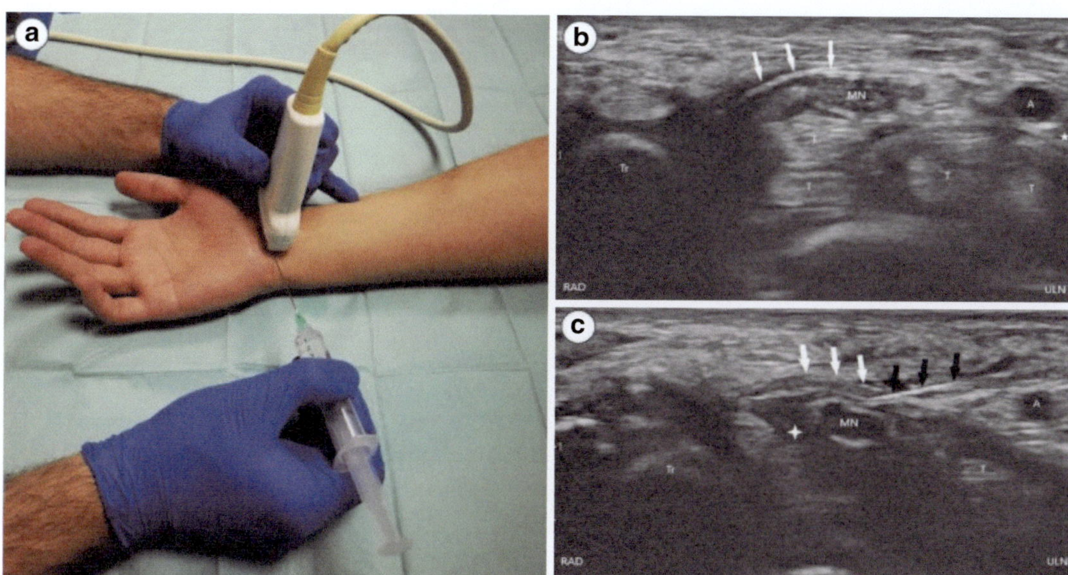

Fig. 3 (**a**–**c**) showing the ulnar approach. (**a**) Wrist and needle positioning for carpal tunnel injection, (**b**) ultrasound anatomy of the carpal tunnel shown in the short axis, (**c**) penetrating transverse carpal ligament positioning the needle tip above the median nerve. Ultrasound of the carpal tunnel after the needle penetrates the transverse carpal ligament. Comparing **b** and **c** note the expansion of the perineural space marked with a white cross (Tumpaj et al. 2022). A = ulnar artery; black arrows = needle; MN = median nerve; RAD = radial; T = flexor tendons; Tr = trapezium; ULN = ulnar; white arrows = transverse carpal ligament; white cross = perineural injectate; white star = ulnar nerve

stiffness or ligament strain from prolonged cross-legged sitting. Regular rest breaks, scheduled every 45–60 min, prevent overuse. Health programs modeled on athletic training, incorporating strength, flexibility, and endurance exercises, are increasingly adopted by music conservatories. Ergonomic practice setups, such as adjustable music stands, supportive seating, or cushioned mats for Indian musicians, and instrument modifications, like lightweight bows or padded drumsticks, reduce strain. For vocalists, vocal hygiene practices—avoiding speaking over background noise, maintaining hydration, and limiting caffeine—minimize laryngeal irritation. Early intervention through routine health screenings and access to performing arts medicine specialists prevents chronicity and supports long-term performance capacity.

6 Objectives of This Book

This book equips clinicians, therapists, educators, and performers with evidence-based strategies to address injuries in musicians and vocalists by:

1. Detailing the epidemiology and multifactorial risk factors of performance-related injuries, including biomechanical, ergonomic, and psychosocial contributors.
2. Exploring diagnostic imaging (X-ray, MRI, ultrasound, laryngoscopy) to achieve precise diagnoses across diverse performer profiles.
3. Presenting evidence-based rehabilitation strategies, integrating physical and voice therapy with ergonomic and psychological interventions to restore function.
4. Promoting prevention through tailored education, health programs, and ergonomic adjustments to minimize injury risk and enhance resilience.
5. Advocating for specialized care and increased awareness to support performers' health and sustain their artistic contributions over longer careers.

By achieving these objectives, *Injuries in Musicians: Imaging and Management* (Table 1) provides a comprehensive guide for clinicians, educators, and artists, advancing the field of performing arts medicine while protecting performers' health and artistry.

Table 1 Summary of common injuries by instrument and recommended imaging

Instrument	Common injuries/disorders	Preferred imaging modality
Violin/Viola	Rotator cuff strain, neck spasm, trapezius myalgia	MRI (rotator cuff), X-ray (cervical spine), ultrasound (shoulder tendons)
Cello/Bass	Thumb tenosynovitis, wrist strain	Ultrasound (tendons), MRI (persistent pain)
Piano	De Quervain's tenosynovitis, carpal tunnel syndrome	Ultrasound (dynamic tendons), MRI (median nerve)
Guitar	Finger joint arthritis, ulnar nerve entrapment	X-ray (joints), MRI (nerve), ultrasound (ulnar groove)
Flute	Wrist extensor overuse, neck pain	Ultrasound (tendons), MRI (cervical spine)
Clarinet/Oboe	TMJ stress, thumb overuse	MRI (TMJ), ultrasound (thumb tendons)
Trumpet	Embouchure fatigue, facial muscle strain	MRI (soft tissue), ultrasound (superficial muscles)
Drums	Wrist tendonitis, shoulder impingement, lower back strain	Ultrasound (wrist), MRI (shoulder/back)
Tabla/Mridangam	Finger synovitis, wrist ligament sprain	Ultrasound (fingers), MRI (wrist ligaments)
Sitar/Veena	Carpal tunnel syndrome, postural low back pain	MRI (spine/median nerve), Ultrasound (carpal tunnel)
Vocalists	Cervical spine strain, TMJ dysfunction	MRI (cervical spine/TMJ), ultrasound (optional TMJ dynamics)

Source: Author (2025)

References

Altenmüller E, Jabusch HC (2010) Focal dystonia in musicians: phenomenology, pathophysiology and triggering factors. Med Probl Perform Art 25(1):3–9. https://doi.org/10.21091/mppa.2010.1002

Baadjou VAE, Roussel NA, Verbunt JAMCF, Smeets RJEM, de Bie RA (2016) Systematic review: risk factors for musculoskeletal disorders in musicians. Occup Med 66(8):614–622. https://doi.org/10.1093/occmed/kqw052

Clemente MP, Mendes J, Vardasca R, Moreira A, Branco CA, Ferreira AP, Amarante JM (2020) Infrared thermography of the crânio-cervico-mandibular complex in wind and string instrumentalists. Int Arch Occup Environ Health 93(5):645–658. https://doi.org/10.1007/s00420-020-01517-6

Kaufman-Cohen Y, Ratzon NZ (2011) Correlation between risk factors and musculoskeletal disorders among classical musicians. Occup Med 61(2):90–95. https://doi.org/10.1093/occmed/kqq196

Kelchner LN, Lee L, Stemple JC (2003) Laryngeal function and vocal fatigue after prolonged reading in individuals with unilateral vocal fold paralysis. J Voice 17(4):513–528. https://doi.org/10.1067/s0892-1997(03)00067-5. PMID: 14740933

Kok LM, Huisstede BMA, Voorn VMA, Schoones JW, Nelissen RGHH (2016) The occurrence of musculoskeletal complaints among professional musicians: a systematic review. Int Arch Occup Environ Health 89(3):373–396. https://doi.org/10.1007/s00420-015-1090-6

Konczak J, Abbruzzese G (2013) Focal dystonia in musicians: linking motor symptoms to somatosensory dysfunction. Front Hum Neurosci 7:297. https://doi.org/10.3389/fnhum.2013.00297

Mangukiya HJ, Kale A, Mahajan NP et al (2019) Functional outcome of De Quervain's tenosynovitis with longitudinal incision in surgically treated patients. Musculoskelet Surg 103:269–273. https://doi.org/10.1007/s12306-018-0585-1

Nyman T, Wiktorin C, Mulder M, Johansson YL (2007) Work postures and neck–shoulder pain among orchestra musicians. Am J Ind Med 50(5):370–376. https://doi.org/10.1002/ajim.20454

Pestana PM, Vaz-Freitas S, Manso MC (2017) Prevalence of voice disorders in singers: systematic review and meta-analysis. J Voice 31(6):722–728. https://doi.org/10.1016/j.jvoice.2017.02.010

Robinson B (2003) Rehabilitation of a cellist after surgery for de Quervain's tenosynovitis and intersection syndrome. Med Probl Perform Art 18:106–112. https://doi.org/10.21091/mppa.2003.3019

Tumpaj T, Potocnik Tumpaj V, Albano D, Snoj Z (2022) Ultrasound-guided carpal tunnel injections. Radiol Oncol 56(1):14–22. https://doi.org/10.2478/raon-2022-0004. PMID: 35148471; PMCID: PMC8884860

Yubran AP, Pesquera LC, Juan ELS et al (2024) Rotator cuff tear patterns: MRI appearance and its surgical relevance. Insights Imaging 15:61. https://doi.org/10.1186/s13244-024-01607-w

The History of World Music: A Global Chronology of Musical Evolution

Akanksh Chokkapu, Urvashi Mohinani, and Indira Guntoory

Contents

A. Chokkapu
Department of Radiodiagnosis, NRIIMS, Visakhapatnam, India

U. Mohinani
Department of Fine & Performing Arts, GITAM, Visakhapatnam, India

I. Guntoory (✉)
Obstetrics and Gynaecology, GITAM, Visakhapatnam, India

Med Radiol Diagn Imaging (2025)
https://doi.org/10.1007/174_2025_629,
Published Online: 26 October 2025

Abstract

This chapter provides a comprehensive chronological exploration of the evolution of world music, tracing its development from prehistoric origins to contemporary digital innovations. It examines music's role as a universal expression of human culture, reflecting societal, spiritual, and technological advancements across diverse civilizations. From the rudimentary instruments of early *Homo sapiens* to the formalized musical traditions of ancient Mesopotamia, Egypt, Greece, India, and China, the narrative highlights key milestones in musical history. This chapter further explores the structural and aesthetic advancements of the Medieval, Renaissance, Baroque, Classical, and Romantic periods in Western music, alongside the distinctive characteristics of non-Western traditions, including Indian classical, Sub-Saharan African, Middle Eastern, East Asian, Latin American, and Indigenous Australian music. The twentieth century's revolutionary shifts, marked by atonality, popular genres, and electronic innovations, are discussed, culminating in an analysis of contemporary trends driven by digital platforms and globalized musical fusion. This study underscores music's enduring capacity to bridge cultural and temporal divides, serving as a dynamic medium for human expression and identity.

1 Introduction

Music, a timeless and transcendent art form, is embedded in the fabric of human civilization. It has evolved in parallel with societies, serving as a vessel for memory, identity, and spiritual expression. From primal rhythms and ritual chants to electronically generated soundscapes, music's trajectory mirrors that of human cultural evolution. This chapter provides a chronological exploration of music's global development, tracing its origins and transformations across epochs and regions.

2 The Origins of Music: Prehistoric Foundations

The genesis of music predates written history, emerging from environmental soundscapes and primitive human communication. Archaeological findings such as flutes fashioned from bird bones and mammoth ivory, dated to over 40,000 years ago, demonstrate early *Homo sapiens*' capacity for complex musical expression (Killin 2018). These instruments, discovered in the Swabian Jura region of Germany, imply a nuanced auditory culture that integrated vocalization and proto-instrumental performance.

3 Music in the Ancient World

3.1 Mesopotamia and the Fertile Crescent

Mesopotamian civilization developed one of the earliest formalized musical cultures. Lyres excavated from the Royal Cemetery of Ur, dating to around 2500 BCE, illustrate music's ceremonial and societal roles (Kilmer and Mirelman 2001).

3.2 Egypt

In ancient Egypt, music permeated both sacred and secular spheres. Harps, lutes, and sistra were widely used in temple rituals and public celebrations. The *Hymn to the Nile* exemplifies the lyrical integration of music into religious practice (El-Malt 2022).

3.3 Greece

Ancient Greek philosophy and aesthetics deeply influenced the theoretical foundations of Western music. Pythagoras is credited with exploring the mathematical structure of harmony and scales, thereby formalizing concepts that underpin Western tonal systems (Crocker 1963).

3.4 India and China

In India, the *Samaveda* provided a scriptural basis for chant and spiritual musicality. Meanwhile, during the Zhou Dynasty, Chinese music emphasized cosmic harmony and moral function, as reflected in the ritual use of bells and guqin.

4 Medieval Music (500–1400 CE)

The medieval period in Europe saw sacred music become predominant, particularly through Gregorian chant, a monophonic vocal tradition standardized by the Christian Church (Daniel 2024). The Notre Dame School in Paris pioneered polyphony, which significantly advanced musical complexity and expressiveness. Simultaneously, secular traditions—propagated by troubadours and minstrels—gained traction across the continent.

5 The Renaissance Era (1400–1600)

The Renaissance marked a resurgence of humanistic values that deeply affected music. Composers such as Josquin des Prez and Palestrina experimented with textural clarity and emotional nuance. The invention of the printing press enabled the mass distribution of musical scores, broadening access and standardization (Cartwright 2020). Secular genres like madrigals and dance music flourished alongside instrumental forms such as those for the lute and early keyboard instruments.

6 The Baroque Period (1600–1750)

Baroque music is characterized by dramatic expressiveness, ornamentation, and the development of forms such as the concerto and opera. Composers including J.S. Bach, G.F. Handel, and A. Vivaldi exemplified the era's aesthetic richness (Encyclopædia Britannica 2025). The introduction of basso continuo and the expansion of counterpoint reflected a heightened complexity in compositional technique.

7 The Classical Period (1750–1820)

The Classical era championed form, proportion, and clarity. Haydn, Mozart, and Beethoven advanced the symphony, sonata, and string quartet, grounding them in balanced melodic and harmonic structures. The growth of public concerts expanded musical access and established music as a central cultural institution (Encyclopædia Britannica 2024).

8 Romanticism (1820–1900)

Romantic music placed emphasis on individual expression, emotion, and nationalism. Composers such as Schubert, Chopin, and Wagner infused their works with narrative and ideological depth. The period also witnessed advancements in instrument construction, enabling richer dynamics and tonal variety (Encyclopædia Britannica 2025).

9 The Twentieth Century: Innovation and Globalization

The twentieth century introduced revolutionary approaches to composition and musical form. Figures like Stravinsky and Schoenberg challenged tonal norms with atonality and serialism. Popular genres, namely, jazz, blues, and rock, emerged in response to urbanization and social change (Baade and Deaville 2016). Electronic instruments and recording technology transformed production and consumption paradigms.

10 Non-Western Musical Traditions

10.1 Indian Classical Music

Structured through raga and tala systems, Indian music emphasizes improvisation and spiritual connectivity. This tradition remains primarily oral, contributing to its fluid and adaptive nature.

10.2 Sub-Saharan Africa

African musical traditions, notable for polyrhythm and communal participation, have influenced genres such as jazz and blues. Oral transmission and drumming ensembles are central to these traditions.

10.3 Middle Eastern Music

The maqam system underlies the modal structure of Middle Eastern music. Instruments like the oud and qanun sustain melodic richness in performance (Encyclopædia Britannica 2011).

10.4 East Asia and Indigenous Australia

East Asian music retains ancient ritual functions, while Indigenous Australian music featuring instruments such as the didgeridoo—encapsulates spiritual connection to land and ancestry (Corn 2013).

10.5 Latin America and Eastern Europe

Latin American music exemplifies cultural hybridity, blending indigenous, African, and European elements. Genres such as samba and tango embody this fusion (Béhague 2024). Eastern European folk traditions use instruments like the balalaika and cimbalom to preserve historical narratives.

11 Contemporary Trends and the Digital Future

Digital platforms have reshaped musical production and distribution, enabling global reach for genres such as hip-hop, EDM, and K-pop. Meanwhile, cross-cultural collaborations and hybrid genres illustrate music's enduring ability to bridge social and geographical divides.

12 Conclusion

The history of music reflects the universality of human creativity. Spanning prehistoric invention to algorithmic composition, music has continually evolved in response to social, cultural, and technological change. It remains a powerful force for expression, identity, and connection across time and cultures.

References

Baade C, Deaville J (2016) Music and the broadcast experience: performance, production, and audiences. Oxford University Press, New York

Béhague G (2024) Latin American Music. Encyclopedia Britannica, 27 February. Available at: https://www.britannica.com/art/Latin-American-music

Cartwright M (2020) The printing revolution in Renaissance Europe. World History Encyclopedia, 2 November. Available at: https://www.worldhistory.org/article/1632/the-printing-revolution-in-renaissance-europe/

Corn A (2013) Sustaining Australia's Indigenous music and dance traditions. Musicol Aust 35(2):268–284. https://doi.org/10.1080/08145857.2013.844526

Crocker RL (1963) Pythagorean mathematics and music. J Aesthet Art Critic 22(2):189–198. https://doi.org/10.2307/427754

Daniel RT (2024) Western Music. Encyclopedia Britannica, 15 March. Available at: https://www.britannica.com/art/Western-music

El-Malt K (2022) Academic study in ancient Egyptian Music. MJAF 7(4):296–304. https://doi.org/10.21608/mjaf.2021.90103.2435

Encyclopædia Britannica (2011) Middle Eastern Music. Available at: https://www.britannica.com

Encyclopædia Britannica (2024) Classical Music. Available at: https://www.britannica.com

Encyclopædia Britannica (2025) Baroque Music. Available at: https://www.britannica.com

Killin A (2018) The origins of music: evidence, theory, and prospects. Music Sci 1. https://doi.org/10.1177/205920431

Kilmer A, Mirelman S (2001) Mesopotamia. Grove Music Online. Available at: https://www.oxfordmusiconline.com

Classification of Non-percussion Instruments

M. S. N. Murthy, Durgananda Lahari Bhamidipaty, Siva Sai Gorle, and Veenadhari Bhamidipaty

Contents

M. S. N. Murthy
Professional Violinist, Visakhapatnam, India

D. L. Bhamidipaty
Department of Industrial Biotechnology, Manipal Institute of Technology, Manipal, India

S. S. Gorle
Department of Radiodiagnosis, NRIIMS, Visakhapatnam, India

V. Bhamidipaty (✉)
Department of CSE, GITAM, Visakhapatnam, India

Med Radiol Diagn Imaging (2025)

https://doi.org/10.1007/174_2025_648,

Published Online: 15 November 2025

Abstract

Non-percussion instruments, encompassing strings, winds, and electronic instruments, form the melodic and harmonic backbone of musical traditions across the globe. Unlike percussion instruments that primarily emphasize rhythm, non-percussion instruments offer a broad expressive range—capable of sustaining tones, shaping melodies, and conveying complex emotional narratives. This chapter delves into the classification, evolution, playing techniques, and acoustical principles behind these instruments. It explores traditional Indian systems such as the *Tata Vadya* (stringed instruments) and *Sushira Vadya* (wind instruments) while drawing parallels with Western counterparts like violins, flutes, and synthesizers. Through a multidisciplinary lens—combining musicology, physics, and cultural history—this chapter offers a deeper understanding of how non-percussion instruments have shaped music across eras and regions. The content is crafted to be accessible yet informative, suitable for readers ranging from students and educators to musicians and enthusiasts.

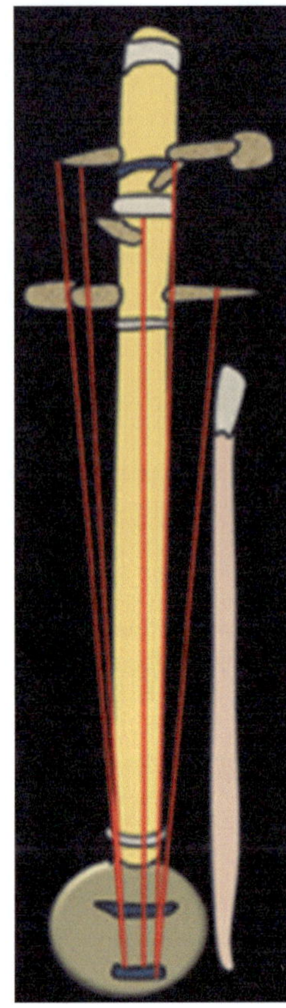

Fig. 1 Ravanastron. (Source: Author)

1 A Journey Through the Strings: A Short History of Stringed Instruments

1.1 The Sound of Strings Begins

Long before orchestras and concert halls, long before pianos and electric guitars, humans were already making music. One of the earliest known instruments with strings—called the *Ravanastron* (Fig. 1)—dates all the way back to around *2500 BC* in Sri Lanka. It was made from a hollow gourd and had a long neck and just two strings. Amazingly, it was played with a bow, much like the violin is today (Westrup 2020). And even more amazing? People still play versions of it today.

Not far away in Mesopotamia, ancient lyres and harps were being crafted and played by hand. These instruments were among the very first to show us how plucked or bowed strings could fill the air with sound—and emotion.

Music was becoming a language of its own, and stringed instruments were right at its heart.

1.2 The Rise of the Bowed Instruments

As centuries passed, these simple stringed instruments evolved. By the *eighth century*, the *rebab* (Fig. 2) appeared—an instrument played with a bow and strung with silk. Its rounded or pear-shaped body rested on the knee or sometimes even had a spike to stand on the floor. Its tuning in fifths made it an ancestor of the modern violin.

By the *tenth century*, more varieties began to appear. Some instruments were plucked, others

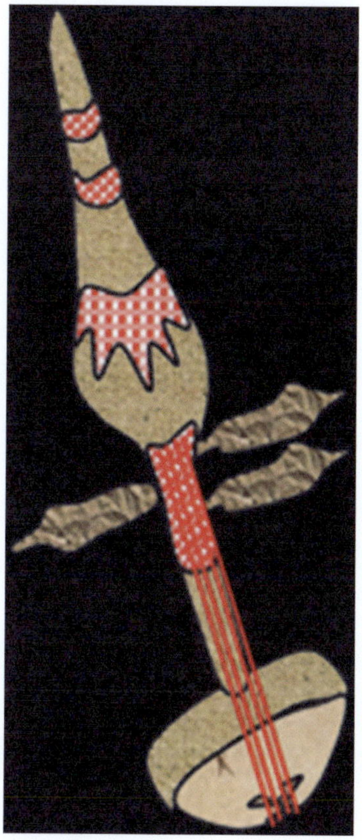

Fig. 2 Rebab. (Source: Author)

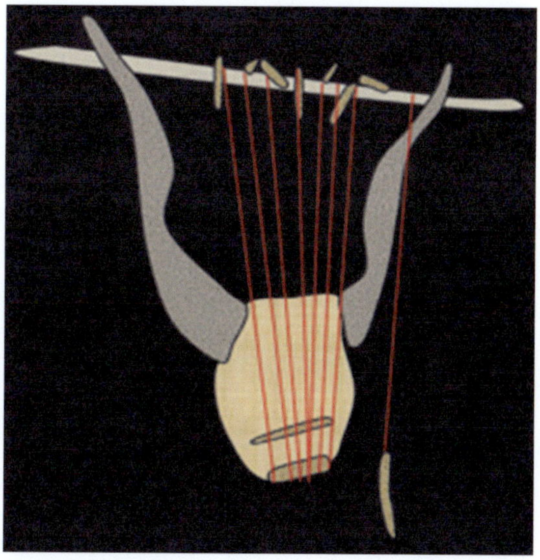

Fig. 3 Lyre. (Source: Author)

bowed. One of the most important was the *viol*, a distant cousin of the violin (Moore 1992; Montagu 2007). These instruments had multiple strings and were played using a bow, paving the way for what we now recognize as the modern string family.

1.3 From Fiddles to Guitars

In the *eleventh and twelfth centuries*, new shapes and styles emerged. The *lyre* (Fig. 3) evolved into what was called the *fiddle*. By the *thirteenth century*, instruments like the *rebec*—with its smooth, rounded body and three strings—were popular all across Europe.

Another instrument gaining fame during this time was the *citole*, a plucked instrument that looked and sounded a lot like today's guitar (Westrup 2020). Music was everywhere: in castles, in villages, and on the streets. Stringed instruments were becoming part of daily life.

In the *fourteenth century*, the *vielle*, also called the Renaissance fiddle, had a body with "C"-shaped sound holes and five strings. The *lute* became the star of the show—the go-to instrument for singers and musicians across Europe. Its gentle, plucked sound became the soundtrack of the Renaissance.

1.4 The European Revolution

Europe played a huge role in shaping modern stringed instruments. Around this time, two new instruments appeared: the *viola da braccio* (played on the arm, like a violin) and the *viola da gamba* (played between the legs, like a cello). These new forms made playing more comfortable and allowed for a deeper, richer sound (Westrup 2020).

Around *1550*, the *first cello-like instruments* began to appear, bringing bass tones into the mix.

Then came a name that would change everything: *Antonio Stradivari.*

1.5 The Master of Strings: Antonio Stradivari

Born in *1644* in Cremona, Italy, Antonio Stradivari became one of the greatest string instrument makers in history. He crafted over *1100 instruments*, including violins, cellos, guitars, lutes, and mandolins. His instruments were not only beautiful in appearance but were prized for their incredible sound.

Stradivari also played a key role in shaping the modern *bow*, giving it the curved, balanced look we still use today.

Even now, centuries later, Stradivari's violins are considered priceless treasures.

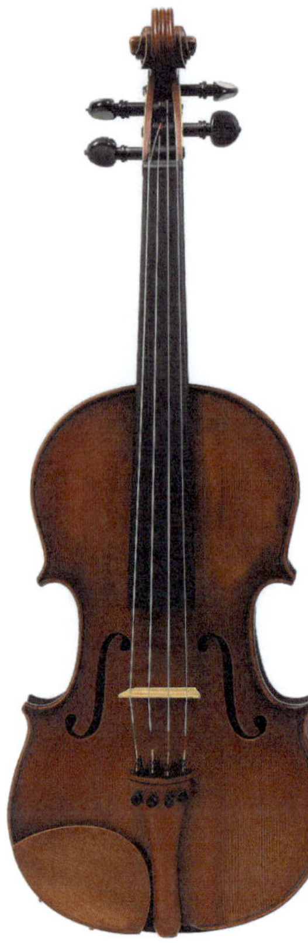

Fig. 4 Violin. (Source: Author)

1.6 The Orchestra Finds Its Voice

By the time *Baroque music* took center stage, string instruments had become essential to orchestras. The core string family we know today was established:

- *Violin* (Fig. 4): the highest voice
- *Viola* (Fig. 5): a mellow middle range
- *Cello*: rich and deep tones
- *Double bass*: the powerful foundation

Interestingly, the *double bass* was not always welcome. It is tuned in *fourths*, unlike the others which are tuned in *fifths*. That difference sparked debate, but in time, the bass found its place as the orchestra's deep, resonant heart.

There was even a bold attempt in the 1800s to go bigger—much bigger. The *octobass* was designed to sound one full octave below the double bass (Moore 1992). The problem: It was so enormous that it was nearly impossible to play. Needless to say, it did not catch on.

1.7 Strings Around the World

While orchestras were forming in Europe, stringed instruments were thriving globally. Instruments like the *guitar* (Fig. 6), *sitar* (Fig. 7), *banjo*, and *mandolin* each followed their own paths in different parts of the world.

These instruments were often the voice of the people—easy to carry, easy to learn, and full of emotion. Folk songs, dances, love ballads, and lullabies were all strummed into being on strings (Kartomi 1990; Lee 2019).

And while the *harp* is used in orchestras (usually with 47 strings and seven pedals!), it is considered a special instrument on its own. The *piano*, despite having over 200 strings, is classified as a *percussion instrument*—because its strings are struck by hammers rather than bowed or plucked.

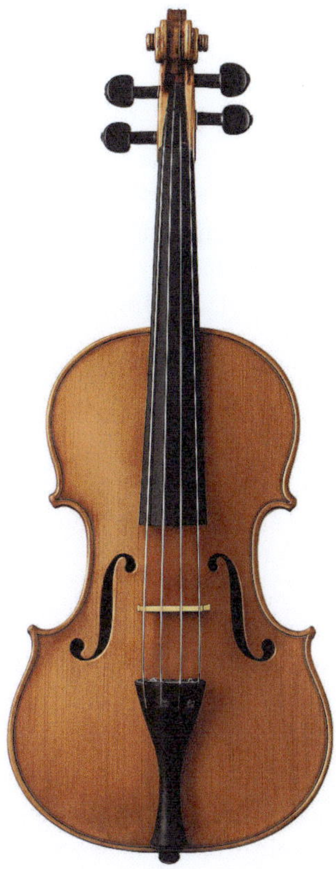

Fig. 5 Viola. (Source: Author)

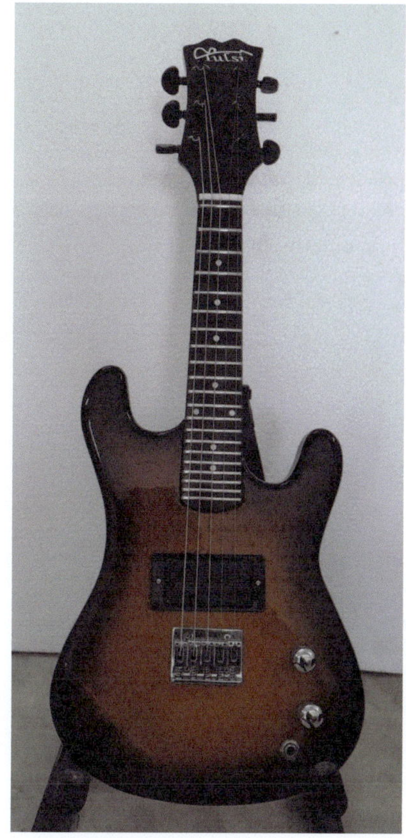

Fig. 6 Guitar. (Source: Author)

1.8 New Materials, New Sounds

For most of history, string instruments used *gut strings*—made from animal intestines. But in the early *twentieth century*, everything changed. Strings made from *steel* and *nylon* became popular. Steel offered a bright, powerful tone, while nylon came closer to the warm, organic feel of gut but was far more affordable and durable (Westrup 2020).

These innovations made instruments easier to tune, more consistent, and longer lasting. It also opened the door to more expressive playing styles and new genres of music.

1.9 The String Goes On

From the Ravanastron to the Stradivarius, from the ancient lyre to the modern electric guitar, the journey of stringed instruments is a story of creativity, craftsmanship, and culture.

Every stringed instrument, no matter how old or new, shares one thing: the ability to touch the human soul. Whether it is a lullaby on a harp, a solo on a cello, or a strum on a guitar around a campfire—strings have always been part of our story (Poudel 2021).

And as music keeps evolving, one thing is for sure: the song of the strings will keep playing.

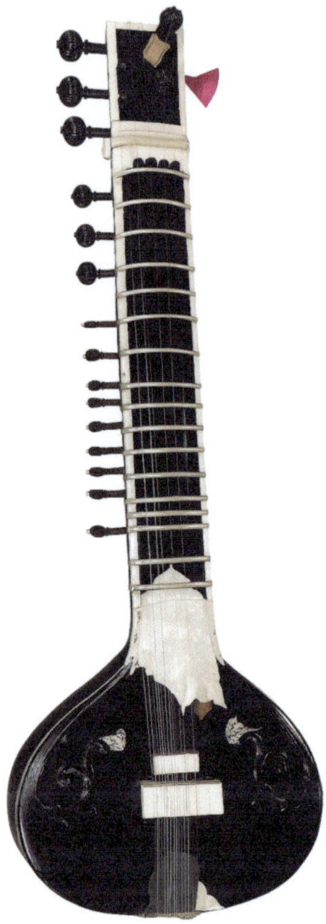

Fig. 7 Sitar. (Source: Author)

2 The Soul of Indian Music

2.1 Introduction: Strings That Tell Stories

In India, music is not just heard—it is felt. And some of the most expressive sounds come from instruments with strings. These string instruments do not just play notes; they *sing*, *weep*, *laugh*, and *tell stories* passed down through generations.

From the northern plains to the southern temples, stringed instruments like the sitar, veena, sarod, santoor, and sarangi have been a part of festivals, prayers, concerts, and quiet practice rooms for centuries.

Let us travel through India's musical heart and meet a few of these amazing instruments.

2.2 The Sitar: The Sparkling Voice of the North

The sitar (Fig. 7) is one of India's most famous musical instruments. With its long neck, curved metal frets, and many shimmering strings, it looks and sounds magical. It is often used in Hindustani (North Indian) classical music and is known for its sweet, echoing sound.

The sitar is played by plucking the strings with a wire pick called a *mizrab*. As the musician gently bends the strings, the notes glide and flow like a river.

Legends like Ravi Shankar brought the sitar to the world stage, and even Western musicians fell in love with its charm.

2.3 The Veena: The Gentle Queen of the South

The veena (Fig. 8) is one of the oldest instruments in India and holds a special place in South Indian (Carnatic) music. It has a wide, wooden body and large round resonators. Its soft, deep sound is like a musical prayer.

Often seen in the hands of Goddess Saraswati, the veena is a symbol of wisdom and learning. It is played by plucking the strings while sliding fingers across the frets, creating a soft, flowing melody (Uddav 2021).

The veena is not just an instrument—it is a bridge between devotion and art.

2.4 The Sarod: The Deep Voice of Emotion

The sarod (Fig. 9) has a smooth, metal fingerboard and no frets, which lets musicians slide between notes effortlessly. Its sound is rich, serious, and full of depth—like someone telling a thoughtful story.

Unlike the sitar or veena, the sarod is played with a wooden pick and uses steel strings. It is mostly heard in Hindustani classical music and is known for its powerful, emotional sound (Poudel 2021).

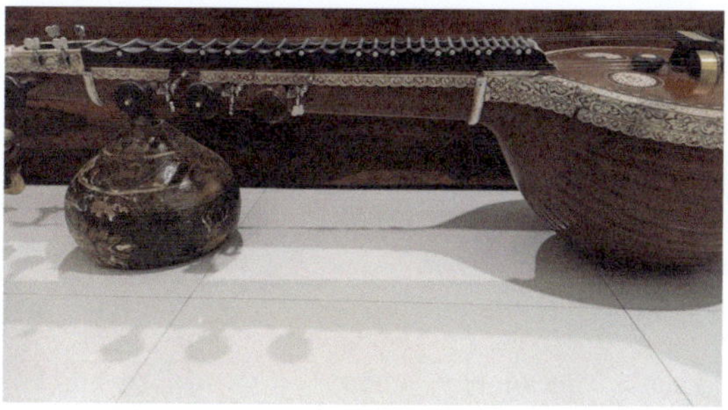

Fig. 8 Veena. (Source: Author)

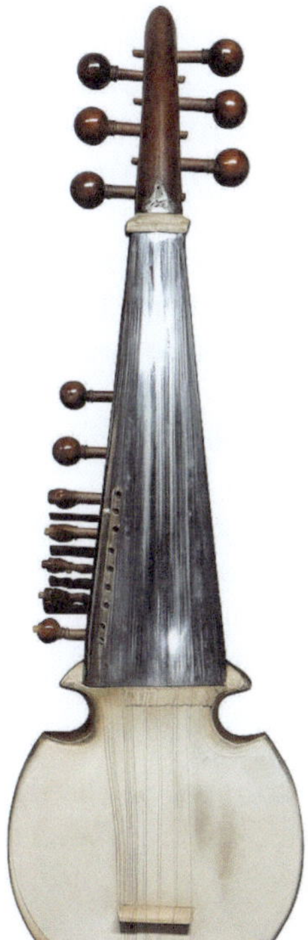

Fig. 9 Sarod. (Source: Author)

2.5 The Santoor: A Box of Bells

The santoor (Fig. 10) is a little different—it looks like a wooden box with many fine strings stretched across it. Instead of plucking, musicians tap the strings with tiny wooden mallets.

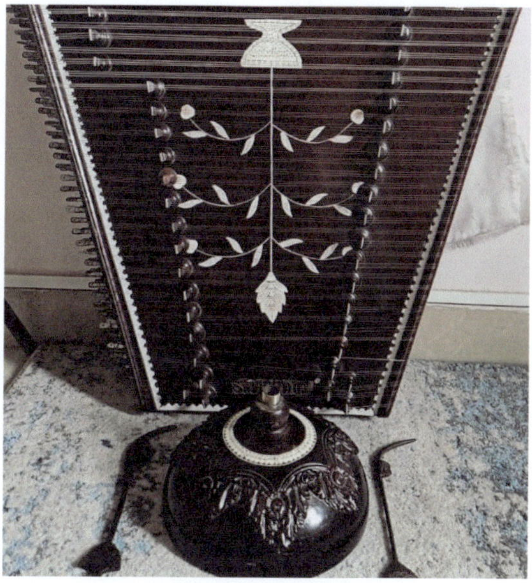

Fig. 10 Santoor. (Source: Author)

The result: A sound like falling rain or dancing light.

It comes from the valleys of Kashmir, where its soft, bright music matches the beauty of the mountains (Poudel 2021).

2.6 The Sarangi: The Voice That Cries and Sings

The sarangi (Fig. 11) is one of the most expressive string instruments in Indian music. Played with a bow, it is said to sound the closest to the human voice. It can cry, laugh, and sing—often all in the same melody.

The sarangi is short and made of wood, with three main strings and many sympathetic strings that add depth and resonance. It is held vertically and played with a bow, while the musician uses their fingers—not to press the strings but to lightly touch them, guiding the pitch with great skill (Moore 1992).

Used widely in Hindustani classical music, as well as folk traditions, the sarangi touches hearts with its raw emotional power.

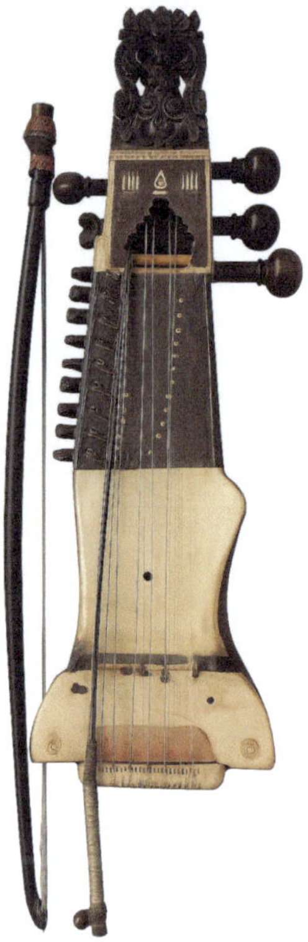

Fig. 11 Sarangi. (Source: Author)

2.7 Bringing It All Together (Table 1)

Each of these instruments comes from a different region, but they all share something special: the ability to speak without words.

- The sitar sparkles with energy.
- The veena whispers with grace.
- The sarod speaks from the heart.
- The santoor dances like wind through trees.
- The sarangi cries and sings like a human soul.

Together, they show how string instruments are more than wood and wire—they are a part of India's voice, echoing through time.

Table 1 Stringed musical instruments and their characteristics

Instrument	Region	Sound character	Played with
Sitar	North India	Bright, echoing	Wire pick (*mizrab*)
Veena	South India	Deep, graceful	Fingers
Sarod	North India	Rich, emotional	Wooden plectrum
Santoor	Kashmir	Light, shimmering	Wooden mallets
Sarangi	North India	Soulful, vocal-like	Bow

Source: Author

3 Aerophones: Instruments of Vibrating Air

3.1 Defining Aerophones and Their Core Principle of Sound Production

Aerophones generate sound by vibrating a column of air, without primary reliance on strings or membranes. A player's breath, a reed, or a sharp edge initiates vibrations, forming standing waves within an air column that produce musical pitches and overtones (Kartomi 2001; Lee 2019).

3.2 Hornbostel-Sachs (H-S) Classification of Aerophones (Table 2)

The H-S system divides aerophones into two main subcategories: free aerophones and non-free aerophones (or wind instruments proper).

Free Aerophones

1. *Displacement-Free Aerophones*: Air meets a sharp edge (e.g., swordblade, whip).
2. *Interruptive-Free Aerophones*: Air stream is periodically interrupted (e.g., accordions, bullroarers).

Table 2 Hornbostel-Sachs subclassification of aerophones

H-S number	Subcategory name	Mechanism/description	Examples
1.	*Free aerophones*	*Vibrating air not enclosed*	*Bullroarer, accordion*
(a)	Displacement-free aerophones	Air meets/moves through a sharp edge	Swordblade, whip
(b)	Interruptive-free aerophones	Air stream periodically interrupted	Accordion, bullroarer, siren
(c)	Plosive aerophones	Single air compression	Thongophone, Udu drum
2.	*Non-free aerophones*	*Vibrating air contained*	*Flute, clarinet, trumpet*
(a)	Edge-blown aerophones	Air stream against an edge	Panpipes, flute, recorder
(b)	Reed aerophones	Vibrating lamella(e) interrupt airflow	Oboe, saxophone (Fig. 12), clarinet (Fig. 13)
(c)	Trumpets	Vibrating lips excite air column	Bugle, trombone, French horn

Source: Author

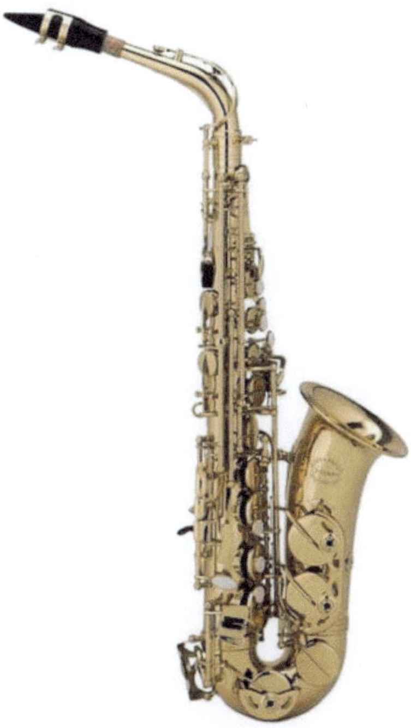

Fig. 12 Saxophone. (Source: Author)

3. *Plosive Aerophones*: Sound results from a single air compression (e.g., Udu drum, Boomwhackers).

Non-free Aerophones

1. *Edge-Blown Aerophones*: Air stream strikes an edge (e.g., flutes, recorders).
2. *Reed Aerophones*: Vibrating reeds interrupt airflow (e.g., oboe, clarinet).
3. *Trumpets*: Player's lips act as a "lip reed" (e.g., trumpet, trombone).

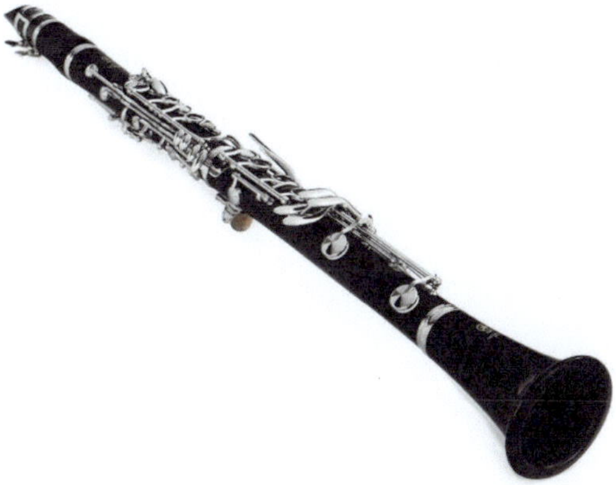

Fig. 13 Clarinet. (Source: Author)

3.3 Acoustical Principles of Wind Instruments

Sound in wind instruments results from vibrating air columns, influenced by bore shape and length. Standing waves form with nodes (minimal displacement) and antinodes (maximal displacement), determining pitch and overtones (Lee 2019).

3.4 Woodwind Instruments (Table 3): Edge-Blown and Reed Mechanisms

1. *Edge-Blown* (*Flutes* (Fig. 14)): Breath directed against an edge causes air column vibration. Pitch is adjusted by opening or closing finger holes, producing a complete harmonic series.

Table 3 Comparative acoustical mechanisms of woodwind and brass instruments

Feature	Woodwind instruments	Brass instruments
Primary vibrator	Air stream or reed	Player's lips (lip reed)
Sound generation	Airflow interrupted by edge/reed	Lip vibrations excite air column
Typical bore shape	Cylindrical or conical	Cylindrical or conical
Overtone series	Complete (flutes, conical) or odd (cylindrical)	Complete (due to bell design)
Pitch change mechanism	Finger holes, keys, overblowing	Lip tension, slides, valves
Timbral qualities	Clear (flute), dark (clarinet), reedy (oboe)	Brilliant (trumpet), mellow (tuba)

Source: Author

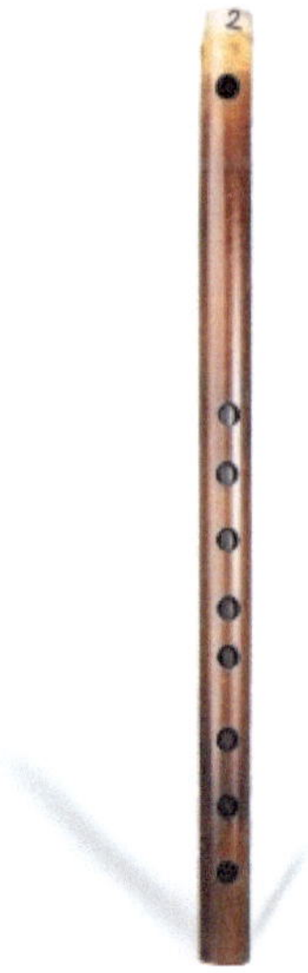

Fig. 14 Flute. (Source: Author)

2. *Single-Reed Instruments [Clarinets]*: A cylindrical bore, closed at one end, yields odd harmonics, creating a "dark" timbre.
3. *Double-Reed Instruments [Oboes, Bassoons]*: A conical bore produces a full harmonic series, contributing to a "reedy" sound.

In summary, bore geometry shapes the harmonic series, influencing timbre and ensemble bleeding.

3.5 Brass Instruments (Table 3): Lip Vibration and Bore Acoustics

The player's vibrating lips act as a "lip reed," exciting the air column. Bore shape (cylindrical or conical) and bell design affect the harmonic series. Cylindrical bores [e.g., trumpet], modified by the bell, produce a complete harmonic series, while conical bores (e.g., tuba) naturally yield a full series, creating a "mellow" sound. Nonlinear wave propagation during loud playing produces the characteristic "brassy" timbre (Herbert 2006).

In summary, lip vibration and bore geometry create brass instruments' distinctive harmonic and timbral qualities.

4 Historical Trajectories and Innovations in Aerophones

4.1 Ancient Origins and Cultural Symbolism

Wind instruments, such as bone flutes from 40,000 years ago, emerged globally for ritual and communication. Ancient Egyptian trumpets and Greek salpinxes served military and ceremonial roles, fostering social cohesion through their loud, symbolic sounds.

4.2 Acoustic Evolution: From Natural Horns to Valved Brass

The nineteenth century introduced valves, patented by Blühmel and Stölzel in 1818, enabling chromatic playing in brass instruments (Herbert 2006). Woodwinds evolved with key systems, such as Boehm's flute design, improving intonation and range.

5 Bowed Chordophones: Instruments of Vibrating Strings

5.1 Defining Chordophones and the Act of Bowing

Chordophones produce sound via vibrating strings, amplified by a resonator. Bowing, using rosin-coated horsehair, creates sustained tones, distinguishing bowed chordophones (e.g., violin) from plucked or struck types (Woodfield 1984).

Table 4 Hornbostel-Sachs subclassification of chordophones

H-S number	Subcategory name	Mechanism/ description	Examples (bowed)
1.	Simple chordophones	Strings on a bearer, resonator not integral	Musical bows, autoharp
2.	Composite chordophones	Integral resonator	Lutes, harps
(a)	Handle lutes	Necked lutes with parallel string plane	Violin, cello, rebab

Source: Author

5.2 Hornbostel-Sachs Classification of Bowed Chordophones (Table 4)

Chordophones include simple chordophones (zithers) and composite chordophones (with integral resonators). Bowed chordophones are classified under handle lutes including the violin family.

5.3 Acoustical Principles of Bowed String Instruments

Sound originates from string vibrations, transmitted via the bridge to the instrument's body. The fundamental frequency depends on string tension, length, and mass, with harmonics shaping timbre.

5.4 The Stick-Slip Mechanism

How does a bow produce a sustained tone? The stick-slip mechanism, as described, involves a rosin-coated bow alternately sticking to and slipping against the string, creating a V-shaped kink (Helmholtz motion) that sustains vibration. Player control over bow speed and pressure shapes timbre.

5.5 Role of the Instrument Body and Resonators

The instrument's body amplifies string vibrations, with the sound post coordinating vibrations between the belly and back plates, ensuring efficient energy transfer and producing the violin's "singing" tone.

5.6 Bow as a Technological Interface: Design and Control

The bow's evolution, culminating in Tourte's 1780s design, enhanced articulation and dynamics through adjustable tension and balanced construction, enabling virtuosic expression (Woodfield 1984).

6 Historical Development and Divergence of Bowed Chordophones

6.1 Early Ancestors and Global Diffusion

Bowed chordophones likely originated in Central Asia (e.g., rebab), spreading to Europe by the eleventh century. Instruments like the rebec and vielle preceded the violin family (Montagu 2007).

6.2 The Violin Family: Innovations and Orchestral Dominance

Andrea Amati standardized the violin's form in the sixteenth century, introducing tuning in fifths and an unfretted fingerboard. Structural modifications, such as a raised bridge, enhanced projection for larger venues.

6.3 The Viol Family: Characteristics and Historical Context

The viol, with fretted strings and a flat back, thrived until the eighteenth century but was overtaken by the violin's versatility. A modern resurgence highlights its historical significance (Woodfield 1984).

7 Conclusion: Intersections and Enduring Significance

7.1 Comparative Understandings of Classification and Sound Production (Table 5)

The H-S system provides an acoustically grounded framework for classifying aerophones and bowed chordophones. Aerophones rely on air column vibrations, initiated by breath, while bowed chordophones use friction-driven string vibrations. Their distinct mechanisms—bore geometry versus stick-slip motion—shape their sonic identities.

7.2 The Enduring Legacy of Aerophones and Bowed Chordophones

From ancient horns to modern violins, these instruments reflect human ingenuity in sound manipulation. Their evolution, driven by technological and musical demands, underscores their role in shaping cultural and artistic expression.

Table 5 Aerophones vs. bowed chordophones: a comparative overview

Feature	Aerophones	Bowed chordophones
Sound source	Vibrating air column	Vibrating stretched string
Initiation method	Breath (edge-blown, reed, lip-reed)	Friction (rosin-coated bow)
Primary acoustic mechanism	Bore geometry, standing waves	Stick-slip motion, Helmholtz motion
Cultural origins	Ancient flutes, ceremonial horns	Central Asian rebab, European violin
Representative instruments	Flute, clarinet, trumpet	Violin, cello, erhu

Source: Author

8 Conclusion

Non-percussion instruments carry the soul of music—where melody takes flight, harmony finds structure, and emotion becomes sound. From the gentle bowing of a violin to the breathy whisper of a bamboo flute or the synthetic hum of an electronic keyboard, these instruments offer an immense range of expression that transcends cultures and eras. They are not just tools for producing music but are extensions of the human voice, echoing our deepest thoughts and feelings.

Understanding non-percussion instruments means appreciating not only their construction and mechanics but also the cultural narratives they embody. Whether rooted in ancient traditions like the *veena* and *bansuri* or thriving in modern orchestras and digital studios, these instruments continue to evolve—bridging the old with the new.

As we conclude, it becomes clear that non-percussion instruments are not merely components of a musical ensemble; they are storytellers in their own right. Their voices, shaped by human touch and breath, remind us that music is both a science and an art, a craft and a calling.

References

Herbert T (2006) The trombone. Yale University Press, New Haven

Kartomi M (1990) On concepts and classifications of musical instruments. University of Chicago Press, Chicago

Kartomi M (2001) The classification of musical instruments: changing trends in research from the late nineteenth century, with special reference to the 1990s. Ethnomusicology 45(2):283–314

Lee D (2019) Music and the science of sound: a guide to instruments of the world. Cambridge University Press, Cambridge

Montagu J (2007) Origins and development of musical instruments. Scarecrow Press, Lanham

Moore G (1992) Nineteenth-century instrumental music. Routledge, London

Poudel R (2021) Indian classical music: tradition and practice. Sage Publications, New Delhi

Uddav S (2021) The veena and Indian musical heritage. Kalakshetra Foundation, Chennai

Westrup J (2020) A history of the stringed instruments. Routledge, New York

Woodfield I (1984) The early history of the viol. Cambridge University Press, Cambridge

Overview of Percussion Instruments and Classification

V. V. R. Murthy, Durgananda Lahari Bhamidipaty, Akeelesh Chengamiah, Siva Sai Gorle, and Veenadhari Bhamidipaty

Contents

V. V. R. Murthy
Professional Mridangist, Visakhapatnam, India

D. L. Bhamidipaty
Department of Industrial Biotechnology, Manipal Institute of Technology, Manipal, India

A. Chengamiah
Department of Music & Dance, Andhra University, Visakhapatnam, India

S. S. Gorle
Department of Radiodiagnosis, NRIIMS, Visakhapatnam, India

V. Bhamidipaty (✉)
Department of CSE, GITAM, Visakhapatnam, India

Med Radiol Diagn Imaging (2025)

https://doi.org/10.1007/174_2025_649,
Published Online: 15 November 2025

Abstract

Percussion instruments are the heartbeat of music. They create rhythm, define tempo, and bring energy and structure to musical compositions across cultures. From the deep resonance of a *mridangam* to the sharp crack of a snare drum, percussion instruments come in countless forms and are found in nearly every musical tradition in the world. This chapter explores the diverse world of percussion—its classifications, cultural significance, playing techniques, and acoustic principles. It delves into both ancient frameworks, such as Bharata Muni's *Natya Shastra* in Indian classical music, and modern systems used globally to categorize membranophones, idiophones, and more. More than just instruments of rhythm, percussion tools are powerful vessels of tradition, communication, and expression. Whether used in rituals, orchestras, or experimental music, their universal presence reveals a shared human instinct to connect through sound. This chapter invites readers to experience percussion not only as instruments but as storytellers that speak through vibration and time.

1 Introduction to Musical Instrument Classification

Musical instruments can be categorized in various ways. In Indian Classical music, the classification suggested by a sage called Bharata Muni in his renowned work *Natya Shastra* is widely accepted (Poudel 2021; Uddav 2021).

2 The Significance of Organology

What links the haunting melodies of a flute to the soaring tones of a violin? Organology, the scientific study of musical instruments, provides the answer by categorizing instruments based on their sound-producing mechanisms (Kartomi 1990). This discipline enables systematic comparisons across diverse musical cultures, moving beyond superficial characteristics like materials or cultural origins.

Organology fosters a deeper understanding of sound production. For example, the shift from colloquial terms like "stringed instrument" to the precise "chordophone" reflects a trend in musicology toward empirical methodologies (Kartomi 2001). This parallels advancements in other humanities fields, where systematic frameworks, informed by sciences such as acoustics, enhance analytical rigor (Lee 2019). By prioritizing universal criteria, organology transcends ethnocentric descriptors, supporting cross-cultural research and interdisciplinary engagement.

3 The Hornbostel-Sachs System: A Foundational Framework (Table 1)

Developed by Erich Moritz von Hornbostel and Curt Sachs in 1914, the Hornbostel-Sachs (H-S) system is the cornerstone of global musical instrument classification (Kartomi 1990; Montagu 2007). Building on Victor-Charles Mahillon's work, it employs a hierarchical decimal notation, akin to the Dewey Decimal System, with five primary categories: idiophones (1), membranophones (2), chordophones (3), aerophones (4), and electrophones (5). This structure facilitates systematic cataloging, supporting ethnomusicological research by providing a universal, expandable framework for analyzing diverse musical traditions.

He divided musical instruments into four groups based on the method of sound production. The four divisions are:

- Tata Vadya—chordophones—stringed instruments
- Sushira Vadya—aerophones—wind instruments
- Avanaddha Vadya—membranophones—skin-covered instruments—percussion instruments
- Ghana Vadya—idiophones/autophones—solid instruments—percussion instruments (Poudel 2021)

Table 1 Overview of Hornbostel-Sachs main categories

Category number	Category name	Primary sound-producing mechanism	Representative examples
1	Chordophones	Stretched strings vibrate	Violins, guitars, pianos, harps
2	Aerophones	Body of air vibrates	Flutes, trumpets, clarinets
3	Membranophones	Stretched membrane vibrates	Snare drums, djembes, kazoos
4	Idiophones	Instrument's solid body vibrates	Bells, cymbals, xylophones
5	Electrophones	Sound produced electrically	Synthesizers, electric organs

Source: Author

The evolution and growth of percussion instruments are deeply interlaced with human history and can rightfully be credited with having a profound impact on humanity (Montagu 2007).

Percussion—the act of striking—was an art in which primitive man was well skilled. The primary roles of early percussion instruments were to accompany dance and support primitive magic and rituals. They held symbolic significance and were believed to possess magical powers. Few instruments were involved in as many ritualistic tasks or regarded as more sacred.

As we can see from the abovementioned classifications, percussion instruments are divided into membranophones and idiophones (Kartomi 1990).

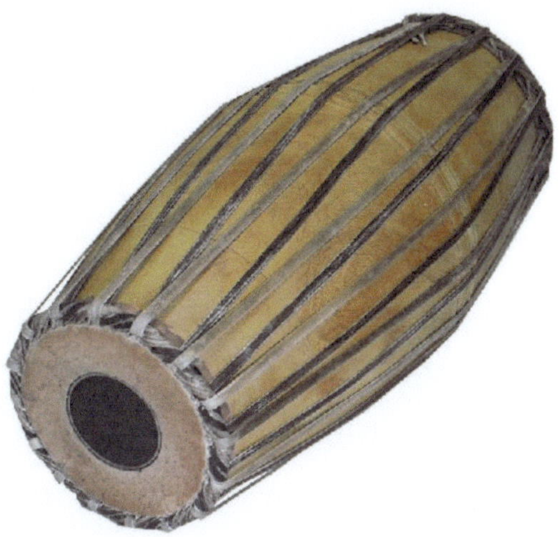

Fig. 1 Mridangam. (Source: Author)

4 Membranophones—Skin-Covered Instrument—Avanaddha Vadya

Membranophones are a category of percussion instruments in which sound is primarily produced by the vibration of a stretched membrane (Lee 2019). These membranes are often made of animal skin or other synthetic materials. We can further divide the classification of the membranophone instruments into instruments being played by hand and instruments being played with sticks.

- Membranophones played by hands: In Indian music, we find instruments such as mridangam (Fig. 1), tabla (Fig. 2), pakhawaj, dholak, and kanjira (Fig. 3); and in other genres of music, we can find instruments such as tambourines, conga drum, djembe, etc.
- Membranophones played with sticks: In Indian music, we can find instruments such as thavil (Fig. 4), idakka, parai, and chenda; and in other genres of music, we can find instruments such as drum sets (Fig. 5) and kettledrums.

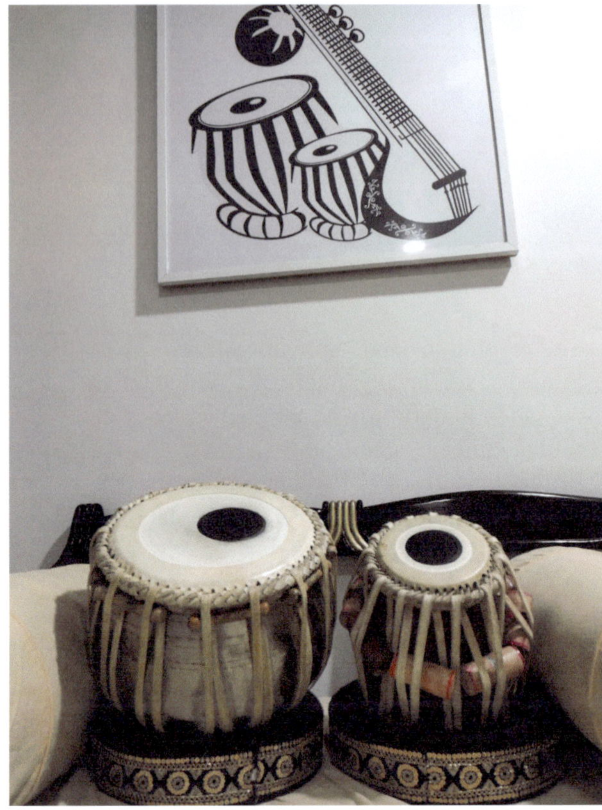

Fig. 2 Tabla. (Source: Author)

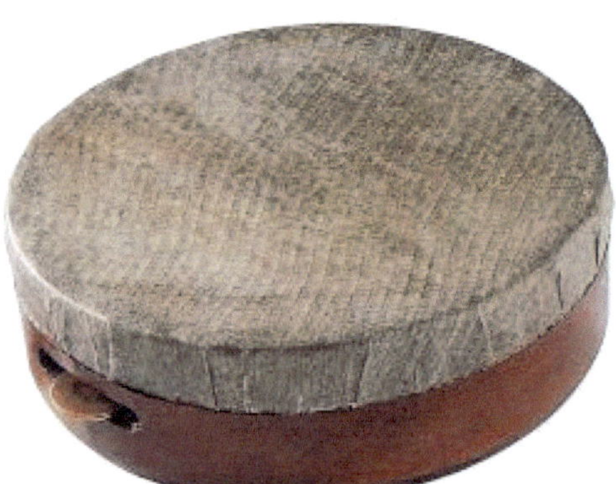

Fig. 3 Kanjira. (Source: Author)

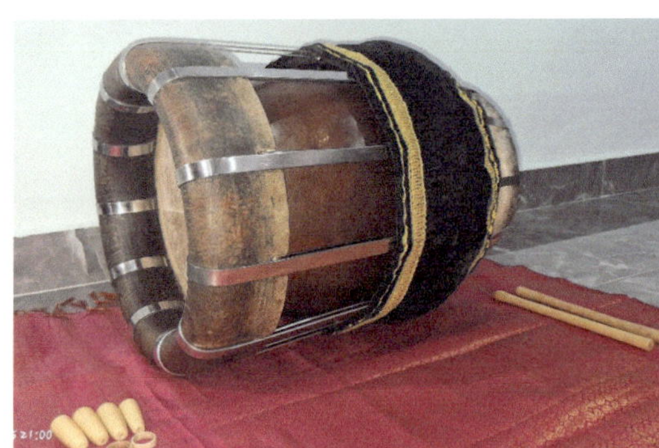

Fig. 4 Thavil. (Source: Author)

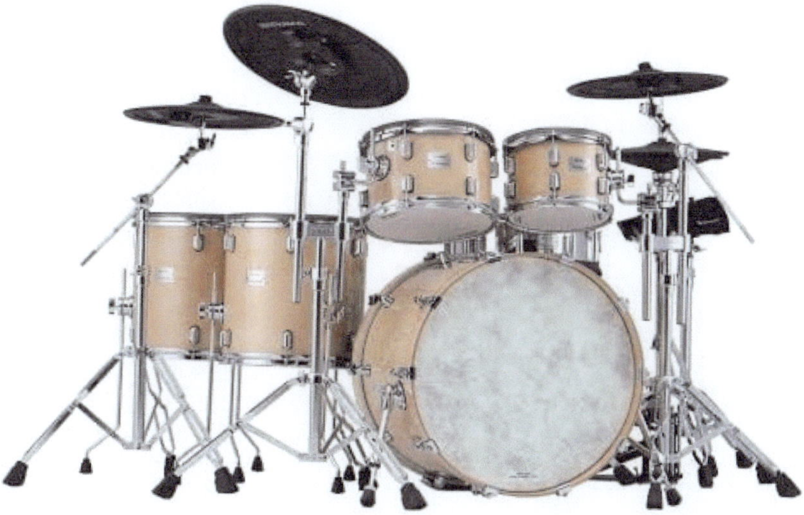

Fig. 5 Drum set. (Source: Author)

5 Idiophones—Solid Instruments—Ghana Vadya

Idiophones are another category of percussion instruments that are produced through the vibration of the body of the instrument (Montagu 2007). Usually, these instruments do not have any membranes, external resonators, or attached strings. They are made of metal, clay, or wood and do not require further tuning.

Examples of idiophones used in Indian music are ghatam (Fig. 6), morsing (Fig. 7), manjira (also known as jalra and kartal), and jala tharang; and in other genres of music, we can find idiophones such as cymbals, xylophones, triangles, etc. (Westrup 2020; Woodfield 1984).

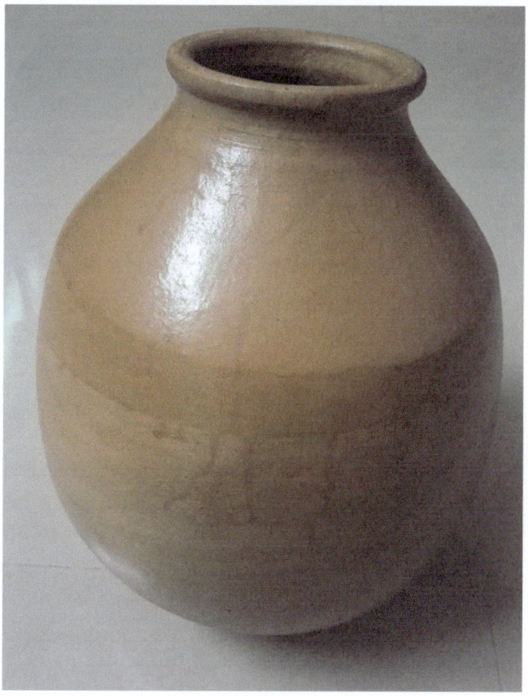

Fig. 6 Ghatam. (Source: Author)

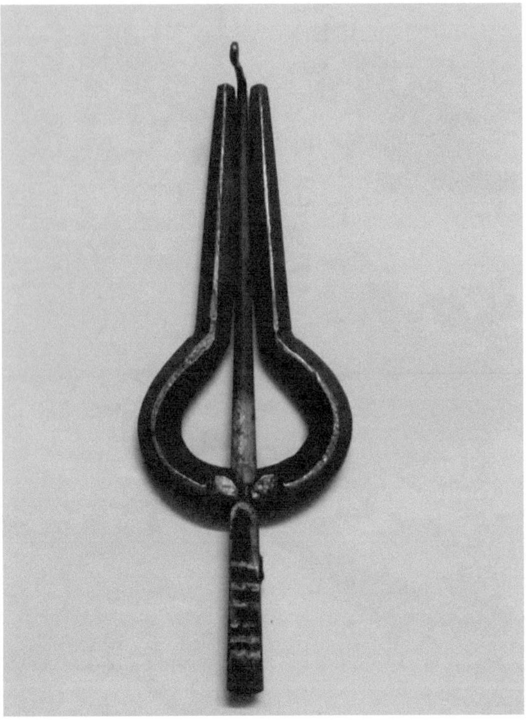

Fig. 7 Morsing. (Source: Author)

6 Role of Percussion Instruments in Musical Ensembles

Percussion is frequently referred to as "the backbones" or "the heartbeat" of a musical ensemble. In almost every genre of music, percussion plays a pivotal role, contributing to the overall rhythm, texture, and dynamics of the performance (Moore 1992; Lee 2019). Some of the roles of percussion instruments are:

- Providing the foundational beat and setting the tempo, ensuring the synchronization among the artists.
- In some genres of music such as symphonies, we can notice that they add intensity and dramatic effects, ranging from soft to powerful climaxes (Herbert 2006).
- Percussion often indicates changes in sections, mood, tempo, and their different rhythmic pattern.
- Percussion instruments sometimes reflect the cultural roots of the music genre, such as the mridangam in Indian classical music or the djembe in African music (Poudel 2021).
- In many musical performances, percussion instruments are given the opportunities for solos to showcase the skills and talents of the performer. For example, in Carnatic music (South Indian classical music), we come across the *Tani Avarthanam,* which allows all the percussionists on stage to showcase their creativity and improvisations, one after the other, by playing a solo.
- In certain genres of music, such as Hindustani music, we can see the pakhawaj and the tabla have evolved and stand as independent solo instruments (Uddav 2021). The artistic depth of these instruments allows performers to showcase their abilities over various compositional forms (*bandish-s*) for extended periods, sometimes exceeding an hour.

Nowadays, because of the diversification of percussion instruments, we can have large musical performances consisting entirely of percussion instruments. We can find rhythm, melody, and harmony in these performances.

7 Biomechanics of Percussion Performance Posture and Playing Techniques Hand, Wrist, and Arm Movements

This research focuses on the posture, playing techniques, and movement of the hands, wrists, and arms of a mridangam, thavil, ghatam, kanjira, morsing, and tabla artist. The biomechanics of percussion performance involve coordination of sitting posture, movements of the hands, wrists, and arms, and playing techniques.
A. *The Posture of a Mridangam Player*

Sitting position A mridangam player's sitting posture is cross-legged on the ground, with the mridangam placed on the right leg. The left leg holds the mridangam as a support, while the right leg is extended to some degree (almost in an "L" shape). The player's hips must remain level to prevent a pelvic tilt.

Description of the sitting posture of a mridangam artist (step-by-step):

- Sit cross-legged on the floor.
- Extend the right leg away from the left leg, creating a gap.
- Place the mridangam horizontally, while the shell of the instruments sits on the right leg. The mridangam is placed usually between the knee and the ankle of the leg, pressing on the calf of the leg.
- The left leg is lifted vertically, while the knee is tucked, and the shin of the leg is pressed on the shell of the instrument creating a support to the mridangam. This will prevent the mridangam from moving.
- The spine of the artist should be straight and relaxed to avoid strain during long practice and performance on stage.
- Shoulders should remain loose, and the neck should stay neutral to avoid any kind of tension.

It is important to note that this sitting posture applies to a right-handed player. For a left-handed player, the same principles apply but in a reversed manner. For instance, the left leg would be extended to create a gap for the instrument, while the right leg would serve as support.

7.1 Hand, Wrist, and Arm Movements

Hand Movements The dominant hand of the artist typically plays the treble side of the instrument. If the artist is right-handed, he/she will play the treble side with the right hand, and if the artist is left-handed, he/she will play the treble with the left hand, producing sharp and rhythmic strokes.

The nondominant hand is used on the bass side of the instrument, producing deeper and more resonant tones.

Wrist Movements Smooth wrist movements are necessary as they help the fingers to reach places on the drumheads easily for efficiency and accuracy and reduce fatigue. To help the fingers navigate easily on the treble head of the instrument, wrist movements such as radial and ulnar deviation movements take place.

Strokes such as *gumki* (bass modulation) involve rolling the wrist subtly to create a characteristic bass effect. Even when practicing strokes such as *tha* and *thom* on the bass head of the mridangam, a lot of wrist extension and flexion take place.

Arm Engagement Arm movement provides power and dynamics, especially during fast sequences or heavy strokes. The movements involve a combination of abduction (moving the arms away from the body) and adduction (bringing the arms back toward the body). Both upper arms are positioned at approximately a 30° angle from the sides of the torso, maintaining a relaxed and comfortable posture.

The forearm used to play the treble head forms a perpendicular angle with the upper arm. This positioning allows the player to strike efficiently, as the treble head is elevated and supported by the right leg. The left arm, which plays the bass head, is kept relatively straight with minimal flexion as the bass head touches the floor. This position ensures precise and controlled strokes on the bass drumhead.

7.2 Playing Techniques

Finger Positioning Various regions of the finger, including the fingertips, middle phalanges, or the entire finger pads, strike the drumhead depending on the desired strokes. It is important to note that strokes are played using either individual fingers (such as *nam*) or a combination of fingers (such as *dhi* on the treble side and *thom* on the bass side), depending on the desired strokes.

Flexion and extension movements of the fingers take place while playing on the treble drumhead of the instrument.

Another crucial aspect of finger positioning is the placement of the thumb. While the thumb is typically not used for playing, its position significantly influences the movement and agility of the other fingers. Depending on the artist's preference, the thumb may rest close to the side of the palm or be held perpendicular to it.

Palm Use The base of the palm is often used to mute or modulate the sound, especially on the left drumhead of the instrument.

Moreover, the shoulders and elbows must remain relaxed, allowing for a smooth transition and reducing tension while playing on the instrument.

B. *The Posture of a Thavil Player*:

There are usually two postures of a thavil artist while playing the instrument:

I. *Seated Posture*: In the seated posture, the thavil player sits cross-legged but extends the right leg forward slightly, creating a gap between both legs. The instrument is placed on the side of the right leg, positioned between the knee and ankle, similar to how a mridangam is held. To maintain stability and achieve a horizontal position parallel to the ground, some artists place a small pillow in the gap to support and elevate the bass side of the thavil.

However, some players just sit cross-legged (lotus posture) and place the instrument in front of them rather than rest it on their leg or lap. The thavil is held closely to the body, with the shell nearly touching the anterior shin splints of the leg. These sitting postures may vary depending on individual playing styles, personal comfort, and the training method by different artists.

II. *Standing Posture*: The standing posture is another common way of playing the thavil, where the player suspends the instrument using a long cloth strap that passes over the shoulder. This allows for mobility, enabling the performer to walk and play simultaneously, which is particularly useful in processions and temple performances.

7.3 Playing Techniques

The thavil is a double-sided drum consisting of a treble head and a bass head.

I. *The Treble Drumhead*: Thavil players usually wear some kind of rings and caps, made of hardened glue using maida flour on their fingers (index, middle, ring, and small fingers) to strike the drumhead, producing a distinctive metallic tone. The drumhead's thick skin makes it impossible to play with bare hands. The playing technique involves flexion and extension movements of the fingers, enabling precise and rhythmic strokes on the treble drumhead.

II. *The Bass Drumhead*: The thavil player uses a stick, known as "kuchi," to strike the bass head. For certain strokes, such as the gumki, the player must slide their palm across the drumhead while simultaneously striking it with the stick. This technique requires radial and ulnar deviation movements of the wrist, allowing for dynamic tonal variations and expressive playing.

7.4 Hand, Wrist, and Arm Movements

Hand Movement The dominant hand of the thavil player is used to strike the treble drumhead, with fingers adorned with rings and caps to enhance the impact and produce a metallic tone. Meanwhile, the nondominant hand holds the *kuchi* (stick) to play the bass head, generating deep, resonant sounds.

Occasionally, the palm of the nondominant hand is rubbed against the bass head while striking it with the stick to create the *gumki* effect, adding expressive tonal variations.

Wrist Movement Wrist movement is important for the nondominant hand, as flexibility and ulnar deviation help guide the stick (kuchi) to strike the bass drumhead effectively. In a standing posture, the nondominant hand's wrist undergoes continuous extension and flexion to maintain control while playing.

Meanwhile, the dominant hand's wrist must remain flexible and fluid, allowing smooth navigation across the treble drumhead for precise and intricate strokes.

Arm Movement In the seated posture, the shoulders remain relaxed, with the upper arms in a natural position and the forearms lifted perpendicular to the upper arms. In the dominant hand, abduction and adduction movements enable the finger caps to strike the treble drumhead effectively. The nondominant forearm also stays perpendicular to the upper arm, with minimal movement.

In the standing posture, the nondominant forearm undergoes significant abduction and adduction movements, allowing the stick to strike the bass drumhead. The nondominant hand is usually kept straight, while the dominant forearm remains perpendicular to the upper arm, executing minimal abduction and adduction movements for precise control over the treble drumhead.

C. *The Posture of a Ghatam Player*

- A ghatam player typically sits on the floor in a cross-legged position (Padmasana/lotus posture) while playing the instrument. Unlike the kanjira and morsing, which are considered as upa-pakka vadyam (secondary instruments in a concert), the ghatam does not need to be held in the hand despite being in the same category.

The player places the ghatam on their lap, positioning the lower round section of the instrument against their thighs while ensuring the mouth (opening) faces the abdomen at a slight angle. Maintaining a straight back is essential, as it allows for free hand movement and better control.

For certain sound modulation effects, particularly the *gumki* (bass effect), the player tilts their abdomen slightly forward, adjusting the angle of the ghatam's mouth to enhance the resonance and depth of the sound. This dynamic positioning enables a wide range of tonal variations and expressive playing.

7.5 Hand, Wrist, and Arm Movements

Hand Movement Both hands are used to play the ghatam. If the player is right-handed, the fingers of the right hand function similarly to those of a mridangam player when playing on the treble drumhead. Additionally, the lower part of the palm or the entire palm is often used in an up-and-down motion to strike the ghatam for the left hand. The tips of the fingers of the left hand are also used for striking specific rhythmic accents on the instrument.

Wrist Movement The right wrist remains flexible and fluid, allowing the hand and fingers to move freely around the ghatam while playing. A flicking motion of the right wrist is used to produce sharp sounds. In contrast, the left wrist is usually held in a more stable posture, as the base of the palm is used to strike the instrument.

Arms Movement The upper arms remain in a natural position, with the shoulders relaxed. The elbows are tucked close to the body, while the forearms are raised slightly upward, allowing the player to strike both around and on the opening of the ghatam. This positioning can be described as a "guard position" for better control and flexibility.

7.6 Playing Techniques

The dominant hand of the player is used to strike the ghatam, similar to how a mridangam player strikes the treble drumhead using their fingers. The distal phalanx of the index finger on both hands is commonly used for striking the ghatam.

Depending on the rhythmic phrase being played, different finger combinations are used. The middle, ring, and small fingers are often struck together, with the entire phalanx of each finger making contact with the instrument.

The ghatam is one of the few percussion instruments where the thumb is actively used.

Typically, on the side of the distal phalanx of both hands, the thumb strikes the ghatam to produce distinct sounds.

On the left hand, the lower palm is primarily used for striking, while the full palm is often applied to the instrument's opening to generate deep bass sounds. Additionally, the fingertips of the left hand play an important role in producing nuanced tones.

Furthermore, the player's abdomen is used to create sound modulation effects, particularly for the *gumki* effect. By pressing and releasing the opening of the ghatam against the belly, the player alters the resonance to achieve this unique tonal variation.

D. *The Posture of a Kanjira Player*

Sitting Position A kanjira player sits cross-legged on the ground, typically in a relaxed lotus posture. Unlike larger percussion instruments like the thavil or mridangam, the kanjira does not need to be secured between the legs or placed on the lap of the performer or the ground. The player keeps a stable posture with aligned hips and an upright back and the shoulders relaxed.

Hand Position The instrument is held in one hand, usually the nondominant hand, while the dominant hand plays by striking the drumhead. The nondominant hand not only holds the instrument but also helps with the modulation of the sound while pressing on the edge of the skin. This technique enables dynamic control over the sound, adding depth and expression to the performance. The Kanjira is a one-handed instrument.

7.7 Hand, Wrist, and Arm Movements

Hand Movement If the player is right-handed, they will hold the instrument in their left hand and play with their right hand. Conversely, a left-handed player will hold the instrument in their right hand and play with their left. While holding and playing the kanjira, both forearms remain perpendicular to the upper arms, ensuring stability and control.

Wrist Movement In the case of a kanjira player, the wrist movement takes place for only the dominant hand engaged in playing on the kanjira, while the other hand's wrist remains stable. Usually, the wrist of the dominant hand moves to help the fingers of the hand reach and strike areas of the drumhead with precision.

Arm Engagement The arm movement is minimal and controlled. The shoulders and upper arms are usually kept still while the forearm of the dominant hand moves in a circular motion to facilitate the drumming.

7.8 Playing Techniques

Finger Positioning The dominant hand strikes the drumhead using different fingers and parts of the palm. Depending on the stroke, various contact points are used, including the entire phalanges of the index finger, finger pads, upper palm, or a combination of fingers to produce distinct sounds on the kanjira.

In addition to the dominant hand, the nondominant hand plays an important role in holding and modulating the sound of the instrument. The thumb rests on the outer rim, while the palm and remaining fingers grip the frame for stability. The palm is placed under the wooden frame, and the fingertips of the nondominant hand press against the skin of the instrument, allowing for precise control over pitch and tone.

Some performer places their thumb on the inside of the frame while the remaining fingers and the palm hold the outer rim of the instrument. Holding the kanjira depends on the individual playing styles, comfort, and training methods.

E. *The Posture of a Morsing Player*

Sitting Position Like any other Indian percussion instrument, the morsing is played while sitting cross-legged on the ground. The player maintains a straight spine, ensuring alignment with the hips while keeping the shoulders relaxed.

Hand Position The morsing is the smallest percussion instrument in Indian classical music, making it easy to hold with the hands. The player uses the nondominant hand (e.g., the left hand) to hold the tail of the morsing. The index finger grips the tail, securing it with the thumb, while the remaining fingers form a fist. Some artists place the index finger on the frame, holding it like a pen.

The morsing is placed inside the player's mouth. Typically, the iron frame (also known as the bridge) rests between the front teeth, though some artists prefer to position it against the teeth while wrapping the lips around it.

7.9 Hand, Wrist, and Arm Movements

Hand Movement The dominant hand (e.g., the right hand) is used for striking. The index or middle finger of this hand plucks the tiny steel reed, which is attached perpendicularly to the central steel rod of the instrument, creating vibrations.

Meanwhile, the nondominant hand, as explained earlier, is solely used to hold the instrument in place inside the mouth.

Wrist Movement The nondominant hand remains stationary, as it is solely responsible for holding the instrument. In contrast, the dominant hand performs repetitive radial and ulnar deviation movements at the wrist, aiding the index finger in plucking the reed of the morsing.

Arm Movement The shoulders remain relaxed, with the upper arms in a natural position. The elbows are tucked in, and the forearms are raised until both hands are near the player's mouth. As a result, minimal arm movement is required to play the morsing.

7.10 Playing Techniques

Plucking Motion The morsing has only a few playing techniques. The player simply needs to secure the instrument between or against the teeth and use the index finger to pluck the small perpendicular steel reed that extends out of his mouth.

Breathing Technique While plucking the reed, the player breathes in and out to sustain the vibrating sound. By rolling the tongue, controlling the throat, and regulating the breath, the player creates different tonal modulations.

F. *The Posture of a Tabla Player*

Sitting Position The tabla player sits cross-legged on the ground with a straight back and relaxed shoulders. The tabla, being a pair of drums, is placed directly in front of the player, close to each other. The drums should be positioned so that they gently touch the tibia (anterior shin) area of the legs and remain centered in front of the body for optimal playing comfort.

Positioning of the Tabla As mentioned above, the tabla consists of two drums: the treble drum, known as the "*Dayan*," and the bass drum, known as the "*Bayan*" or "*Dagga*." For right-handed performers, the *Dayan* is placed on the right side and the *Bayan* on the left. Conversely, for left-handed performers, the *Dayan* is placed on the left, while the *Bayan* is on the right. To prevent the instrument from moving, each drum is placed on a round-shaped cushion called "*Indri*."

Hand Position Both hands are used to play the tabla. The player should position their hands on each drum, ensuring a comfortable reach. The arms should remain relaxed, avoiding any stiffness.

Moreover, the shoulders should be kept level to maintain balance and prevent strain.

7.11 Hand, Wrist, and Arm Movements

Hand Movement For a right-handed player, the dominant right hand is used to play the *Dayan*, while the left-hand plays the *Bayan*. Conversely, for a left-handed player, the left hand plays the *Dayan*, and the right hand plays the *Bayan*.

Wrist Movement Similar to the mridangam, smooth wrist movements are essential for allowing the fingers to reach different areas of the tabla drumheads. On the dominant hand, the wrist undergoes radial and ulnar deviation, enabling the execution of various strokes with ease. On the nondominant hand, the wrist performs extension and flexion movements to produce sound modulation syllables such as *Ge* (equal to the *gumki* syllable on the mridangam) and *Ke* (a single slap on the *Bayan*) on the bass drumhead.

Arms Movement The shoulders and elbows should remain relaxed, with the shoulders kept low to avoid tension. The upper arms should be in a natural position, ensuring that the elbows are not too close to the body. Most of the movement should come from the wrists rather than the arms.

7.12 Playing Techniques

Finger Positioning On the dominant hand, all four fingers (index, middle, ring, and little finger) are used to strike different areas of the drumhead. The index finger strikes with either the distal phalanx or the entire phalanx to produce syllables like *Nam* and *Tin*. In contrast, the other three fingers use only the distal phalanx to produce strokes such as *Ti* and *Te*.

The thumb is generally not used for striking but plays a supportive role, assisting the other fingers and providing stability.

On the *Bayan*, the fingertips are used to produce strokes like *Ge*. Typically, the tip of the index finger and the tip of the middle finger (often joined with the ring finger) strike the drumhead to generate the bass sound.

Palm To modulate the sound of the syllable *Ge*, the player must slide or press the wrist crease of their nondominant hand on the *Bayan* to create the desired bass effect.

For syllables like *Ke*, the player strikes the *Bayan* using the full palm and fingers, keeping them flat against the drumhead.

The palm is also used on the dominant hand while playing *Dhere Dhere* on the *Dayan*. The player first strikes with the right side of the palm (just below the little finger), followed by the left side of the palm (near the base of the index finger).

8 Conclusion

Percussion instruments are more than just timekeepers—they are the pulse of music, the primal echo of the human spirit. Whether it is the steady beat of a drum in a folk festival, the intricate rhythm of a tabla solo in a classical concert, or the explosive cadence of a marching band, percussion speaks a language that everyone can feel, even without words.

Throughout history and across cultures, these instruments have served as both musical foundations and emotional catalysts. They signal celebration, mark sacred rituals, and drive the dynamics of every ensemble. Their variety—ranging from simple clappers to sophisticated tuned percussion—reflects the creativity and diversity of human expression.

As we conclude this exploration, one truth stands clear: percussion instruments connect us to our roots, to each other, and to the heartbeat of the music itself. They remind us that rhythm is not just an element of sound—it is a reflection of life, movement, and the shared pulse of humanity.

References

Herbert T (2006) The trombone. Yale University Press, New Haven

Kartomi M (1990) On concepts and classifications of musical instruments. University of Chicago Press, Chicago

Kartomi M (2001) The classification of musical instruments: changing trends in research from the late nineteenth century, with special reference to the 1990s. Ethnomusicology 45(2):283–314

Lee D (2019) Music and the science of sound: a guide to instruments of the world. Cambridge University Press, Cambridge

Montagu J (2007) Origins and development of musical instruments. Scarecrow Press, Lanham

Moore G (1992) Nineteenth-century instrumental music. Routledge, London

Poudel R (2021) Indian classical music: tradition and practice. Sage Publications, New Delhi

Uddav S (2021) The veena and Indian musical heritage. Kalakshetra Foundation, Chennai

Westrup J (2020) A history of the stringed instruments. Routledge, New York

Woodfield I (1984) The early history of the viol. Cambridge University Press, Cambridge

Injuries Specific to Vocal Music and Radiological Features

Suhel Hasan, Smita Caren Mathias, Muralidhar K., and Kanaka Durga Prasad Bhamidipaty

Contents

Abstract

Singing is a powerful form of expression, but behind the beauty of the human voice lies a complex physical effort that can sometimes lead to injury. Vocalists, especially professionals, often push their voices to the limit—sometimes without realizing the strain it causes. This chapter delves into the common injuries faced by singers, such as vocal nodules, polyps, swelling, or strain in the vocal cords. We explore how these conditions arise, from overuse, poor technique, or even emotional tension, and how they can affect a singer's performance and well-being.

We also look at how modern imaging techniques—like laryngoscopy, stroboscopy, ultrasound, and MRI—help in identifying and understanding these injuries. These tools give us a window into the voice box and help clinicians provide the right treatment. By combining medical insight with practical knowledge of the singing profession, this chapter aims to support both vocalists and voice care professionals in preventing injuries and promoting long-term vocal health.

The original version of this chapter was revised. The omitted co-authors have been included in the author byline. A correction to this chapter can be found at https://doi.org/10.1007/978-3-032-14365-5_658

S. Hasan
Department of ENT, Mazumdar Shaw Medical Centre, Narayana Health, Bengaluru, India

S. C. Mathias
Speech Language Pathology and Deglutology, Society for Feeding and Swallowing Disorders, (SFSD) India, Narayana Health City, Bengaluru, India

Muralidhar K.
Department of Anaesthesia, Narayana Hrudayalaya Hospital, Bangalore, India

K. D. P. Bhamidipaty (✉)
Department of Radiodiagnosis, NRIIMS, Visakhapatnam, India

Med Radiol Diagn Imaging (2025)

https://doi.org/10.1007/174_2025_631,
corrected publication 2026
Published Online: 26 October 2025

1 Introduction

Vocal music, an art form that relies on the human voice as its primary instrument, requires a delicate balance between vocal technique, physical health, and mental well-being. Singers are specialized voice users with or without formal vocal training, ranging from amateur singers who sing primarily for enjoyment to semi-professional and professional singers who perform for monetary benefits. They are sometimes referred to as vocal athletes because of their higher phonatory agility, stamina, and strength, enabling the production of superior vocal quality, pitch, and loudness (Kwok and Eslick 2017). When singing, vocalists rely on complex interactions between their respiratory system, laryngeal muscles, and other structures within the vocal tract (Arunachalam et al. 2014). Professionals need to maintain their vocal quality during their performances which requires intense vocal effort. Given the physical demands of singing, vocalists can be susceptible to a range of vocal injuries. Even minor issues, which may be imperceptible or insignificant to others, may produce a profound impact on the vocal performance. These injuries may occur as a result of improper technique, overuse, or a lack of proper vocal care. Understanding the causes, types, and treatments of vocal injuries is crucial for both aspiring and professional vocalists to maintain long-term vocal health.

This chapter will explore the types of injuries that vocalists can experience, their causes, symptoms, and treatment options. Furthermore, it will examine preventative measures and the role of vocal training in reducing the risk of injuries. Through a combination of medical knowledge, vocal pedagogy, and research from various sources, this chapter aims to provide a comprehensive overview of vocal injuries in singers.

2 Anatomy of the Voice

To understand the mechanisms behind vocal injuries, it is essential to first examine the anatomy and physiology of the voice. Sound generation of any type requires a (1) power source, (2) vibrator, and (3) resonator: the *lungs* are the power supply, the *larynx* is the vibratory source, and the *supraglottal vocal tract* —supraglottic larynx, pharynx, oral cavity, and, potentially, the nasal cavity—is the resonator, which shapes the sound into words and song.

1. Lungs and diaphragm: The lungs provide air that is pushed out by the diaphragm to produce sound. The diaphragm, a large muscle beneath the lungs, controls airflow and breath support for singing.
2. Larynx and vocal folds: The larynx, or voice box, houses the vocal folds. When air passes through the trachea into the larynx, the vocal folds vibrate, creating sound. The tension and position of the vocal folds are controlled by intrinsic muscles of the larynx, allowing for variations in pitch, loudness, and quality of sound. The extrinsic laryngeal muscles alter the position of the larynx, which, in turn, can affect the length of the vocal tract resonator. Classically trained singers use the extrinsic musculature to stabilize the larynx within the neck when singing.
3. Resonating cavities: The sound produced in the larynx is then modified by the resonating spaces of the throat, mouth, and nasal passages. These cavities amplify and shape the sound, contributing to the unique timbre of the voice.
4. Breathing coordination: Singing requires coordinated breath control, which ensures the smooth transition from inhaling to exhaling and vocalizing. Effective control of air pressure and release is fundamental to healthy vocal production.

Understanding this system is key to recognizing how misuse or strain on any of these components can lead to injury.

3 Neurologic Control of Voice

The external and muscles of larynx are supplied by the vagus nerve which is responsible for their complex coordinated movements producing voice.

Sensory and motor innervation of the larynx is by two branches of the vagus nerves [X]—the superior laryngeal nerves and the recurrent laryngeal nerves.

I. Superior laryngeal nerves: The superior laryngeal nerves in turn divide into internal and external laryngeal nerves on each side.
   - The external laryngeal nerve penetrates the inferior constrictor of the pharynx and ends by supplying the cricothyroid muscle.
   - The internal laryngeal nerve passes antero-inferiorly to penetrate the thyrohyoid membrane—it is mainly sensory and supplies the laryngeal cavity down to the level of the vocal folds.

II. Recurrent laryngeal nerves: The recurrent laryngeal nerves provide sensory supply to the laryngeal cavity below the level of the vocal folds, and motor supply to all intrinsic muscles of the larynx except for the cricothyroid (Drake et al. 2014).

4 Physiology of Voice

In 1974, Hirano published the *cover-body theory* of vocal fold vibration. He divided the vocal folds biomechanically into the body and the cover layer. The main substance of the vocal fold is the thyroarytenoid (TA) muscle *(body)*. Overlying the TA is vocal ligament. Superficial to the body lies the vocal fold epithelium and superficial layer of the lamina propria loosely associated with the vocal ligament. The superficial lamina propria and epithelium move as a vibratory unit (*cover*) weakly coupled to the body. Therefore, this *cover-body theory* of vocal fold vibration dictates the vocal folds function at least as a double-structured vibrator. The tissue of the vocal fold is displaced in a wave-like fashion, creating the so-called mucosal wave. Because the mucosal wave is dependent on vocal fold structure, physical alterations of that structure cause mucosal wave abnormalities (Wang et al. 2021).

Fundamental frequency (F_0) is the number of repeating cycles per second present in the acoustic waveform. The average speaking fundamental frequency ranges from 100 to 125 Hz for adult men and 190 to 225 Hz for adult women. Pitch is the primary perceptual correlate of frequency. Changes in vocal fold length and tension are used to control the fundamental frequency of vocal fold vibration, thereby increasing or decreasing the pitch. This requires fine motor control which is very essential for singing (Wang et al. 2021).

5 Types of Vocal Injuries

Vocal injuries in singers can range from minor irritations to serious, long-term damage. The most common injuries include vocal fold nodules, polyps, cysts, muscle tension dysphonia, and laryngitis.

1. *Vocal Fold Nodules*: Vocal nodules are defined as bilateral symmetric epithelial swelling of the anterior/mid third of the true vocal folds due to repeated trauma or overuse. These nodules are often compared to calluses on a finger, as they form from consistent friction during phonation (sound production). They range from soft vocal fold swellings without fibrous duplication of the underlying stroma to hard keratinized nodule. Nodules typically appear on the middle portion of the vocal folds and can cause hoarseness, breathiness, or a reduced vocal range.
   Causes: Phonotrauma such as overuse of the voice, improper vocal technique, or excessive loud singing. It is especially common in singers who sing at the top of their range or who push their voices beyond their natural limits. The pathophysiology of vocal nodules relies on the mid-membranous vocal fold experiencing maximal shearing and collision forces. This location corresponds to the junction of the anterior to middle vocal folds (because the posterior third of the vocal folds is coupled to the vocal process of the arytenoids). This repeated collision initially results in localized vascular congestion with edema. Eventually hyalinization of Reinke space with thickening of overlying epithelium

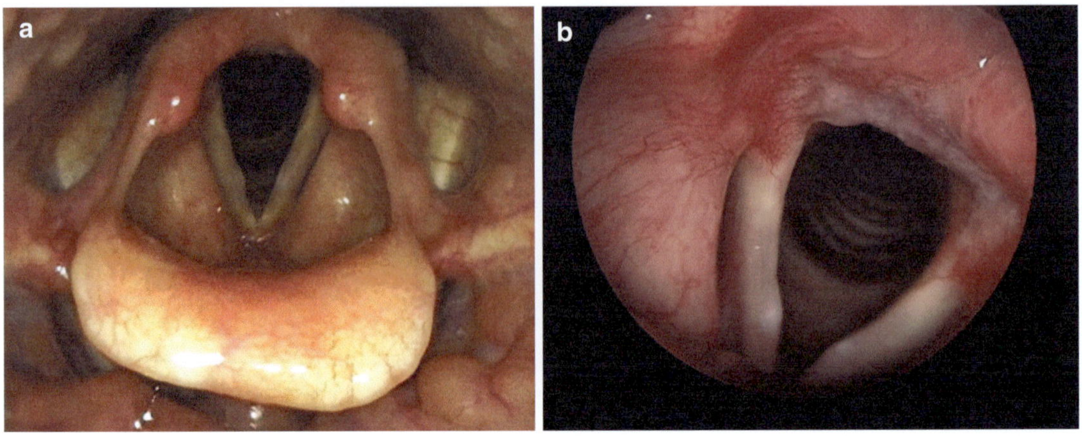

Fig. 1 Video-laryngoscopic images showing bilateral vocal cord nodules (**a**) with stroboscopy (**b**) without stroboscopy

occurs with the development of epithelial hyperplasia (Altman 2007).

(i) Symptoms: Hoarseness, vocal fatigue, and discomfort while singing or speaking, throat dryness, or tightness, reduced vocal range, and vocal fatigue. Singers may experience difficulty reaching higher notes or a scratchy voice.

(ii) Videostroboscopy: Strobolaryngoscopy reveals bilateral symmetric superficial swelling of the vocal folds at the striking zone junction of the anterior to middle thirds (Fig. 1). There is slightly decreased amplitude of the mucosal wave, but the wave is generally symmetric.

(iii) Treatment: The main line of treatment of nodules is conservative management in the form of voice therapy, voice rest, and vocal hygiene. Most voice therapy programs usually last 6–12 weeks. Surgical excision of nodules is another treatment option; however, it is usually done after the failure of conservative management. Vocal fold steroid injection (VFSI) may also be attempted which acts by reducing inflammation.

2. Vocal Polyps

Vocal polyps are soft, fluid-filled growths that occur on one or both vocal folds. Unlike nodules, polyps are more like blisters and can vary in size. They can result from a single traumatic event, such as shouting or singing loudly without proper technique.

(i) Causes: Polyps can develop after a single instance of vocal trauma or from chronic vocal strain, laryngopharyngeal reflux, *H. pylori* infection, and smoking. The pathophysiology is believed to be attributable to breakage of a capillary in Reinke space (superficial lamina propria) with subsequent extravasation of blood, resultant local edema, and ultimate organization with hyalinized stroma. The resulting mass may be broad-based or pedunculated, and hemorrhagic versus nonhemorrhagic (Altman 2007).

(ii) Symptoms: A hoarse or raspy voice, difficulty singing high notes, or a feeling of a "lump" in the throat. Some singers may also experience vocal fatigue and discomfort.

(iii) Videostroboscopy: On strobolaryngoscopy, vocal folds with small polyps generally have intact mucosal waves but phase asymmetry because of the impaired phase closure and the mass effect of the polyp (Figs. 2 and 3). Vocal folds with larger polyps have more prominent decreased mucosal wave amplitude.

(iv) Treatment: Treatment may involve voice rest, vocal therapy, and surgery to remove the polyp. Surgery includes phonomicro-

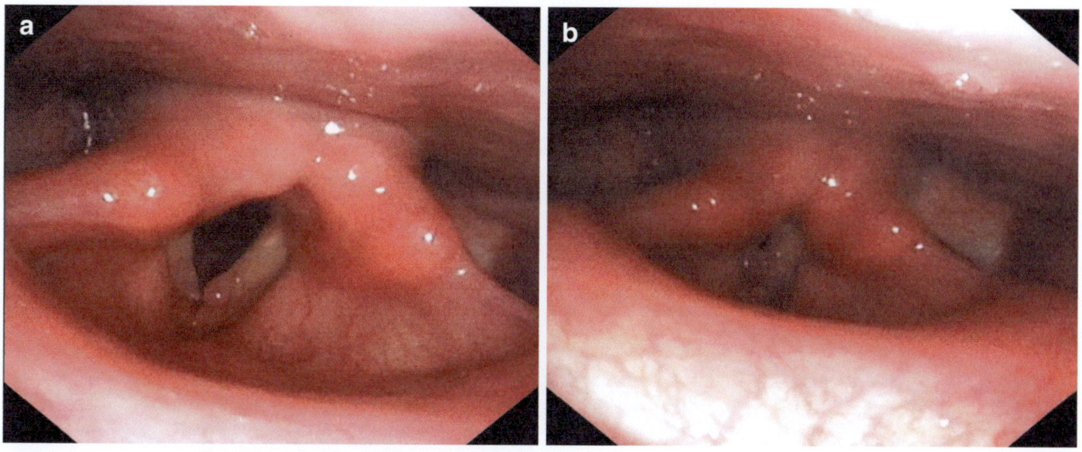

Fig. 2 Video-laryngoscopic images showing bilateral vocal cord polyp (**a**) in abduction (**b**) in adduction

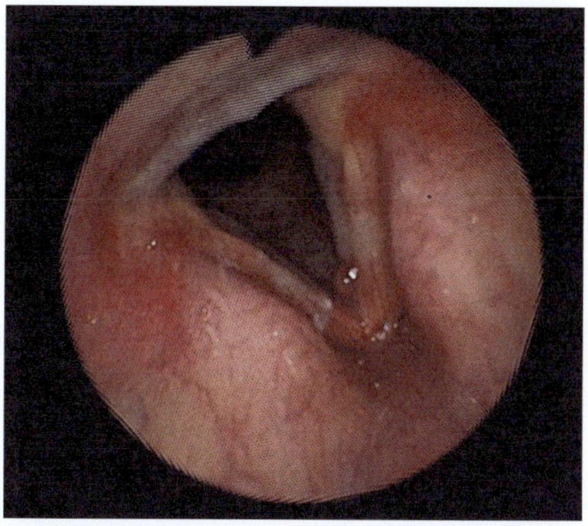

Fig. 3 Video-laryngoscopic images showing left vocal cord polyp

surgery, angiolytic laser, and subepithelial steroid injection. Recovery may require changes to singing technique to prevent recurrence.

3. Vocal Cysts

Cysts are subepidermal epithelial-lined sacs located within the lamina propria and may be mucus retention or epidermoid in origin. Mucus retention cysts form when a mucous gland duct becomes obstructed (usually during an upper respiratory infection or with overuse), retaining glandular secretions. Epidermoid cysts develop either from congenital cell rests in the subepithelium of the fourth and sixth branchial arches or from healing injured mucosa burying epithelium.

(i) Causes: Chronic misuse or overuse of the voice, such as in singers who habitually push their vocal folds beyond their natural limits. Vocal limitation is less than expected from its size.

(ii) Symptoms: Hoarseness, difficulty controlling pitch, and a reduced ability to sing high notes. Cysts can also cause a "breathy" quality in the voice.

(iii) Videostroboscopy: On strobolaryngoscopy, the vocal folds appear asymmetric with occasional evidence of the subepithelial mass (Fig. 4). Because of displacement of lamina propria, there is significant decreased or absent mucosal wave on the side of the cyst.

(iv) Treatment: Surgical removal is often required to treat vocal cysts, followed by voice rest and rehabilitation to prevent recurrence. A true cyst does not resolve with conservative management. Leaving behind a minute fragment of epithelium in the cyst sac may result in recurrence of the cyst. Hence, it requires more extensive dissection because the cyst is in the submucosal plane.

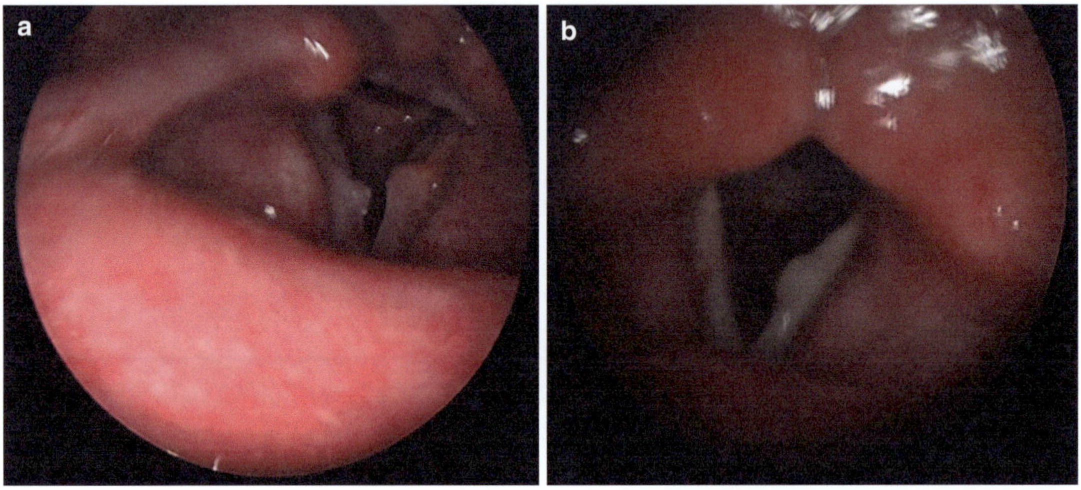

Fig. 4 Video-laryngoscopic images showing (**a**) bilateral vocal cord cysts (**b**) left-sided vocal cord cyst

4. Muscle Tension Dysphonia (MTD)
   Muscle tension dysphonia occurs when the muscles around the larynx (such as the neck, jaw, and throat muscles) become tense and overactive, leading to strain and discomfort during speaking or singing. This condition often results from poor posture, anxiety, or incorrect vocal technique.
   (i) Causes: Stress, emotional strain, poor vocal habits, and improper technique can all contribute to MTD.
   (ii) Symptoms: Vocal fatigue, hoarseness, tension in the neck or throat, and discomfort while speaking or singing. Singers may find it difficult to sing without effort, and the voice may sound strained or tight.
   (iii) Treatment: Voice therapy with an SLP, relaxation techniques, and awareness of posture can be beneficial in alleviating the symptoms of MTD.
5. Laryngitis
   Laryngitis is the inflammation of the larynx (voice box) often caused by viral infections, bacterial infections, overuse of the voice, or exposure to irritants like smoke or pollutants. It is a common condition among singers and speakers (Fig. 5).
   (i) Causes: Viral infections (such as the common cold), excessive voice use (such as shouting or loud singing), exposure to irritants, or dehydration. Inflammation of the vocal folds causes irritation and edema and hinders the pliable motion of the mucosa, which leads to dysphonia. To compensate, singers may exert extra effort to maintain the normal voice.
   (ii) Symptoms: Hoarseness, a dry or scratchy throat, reduced vocal range, and vocal fatigue.
   (iii) Treatment: Preferred management of laryngitis involves an increase in fluid intake and humidification of the room. If a cough is present, an antitussive agent may be of benefit; however, conservative voice use is key so the singer should speak little, if at all, to allow the vocal folds to heal. Before the performance, the singer should warm up in a normal fashion and should be told not to force the voice to produce the usual or normal sound. The performer should be instructed to sing by feel and not by sound because this technique may avoid exacerbating the injury. The singer should speak in a normal, unforced voice

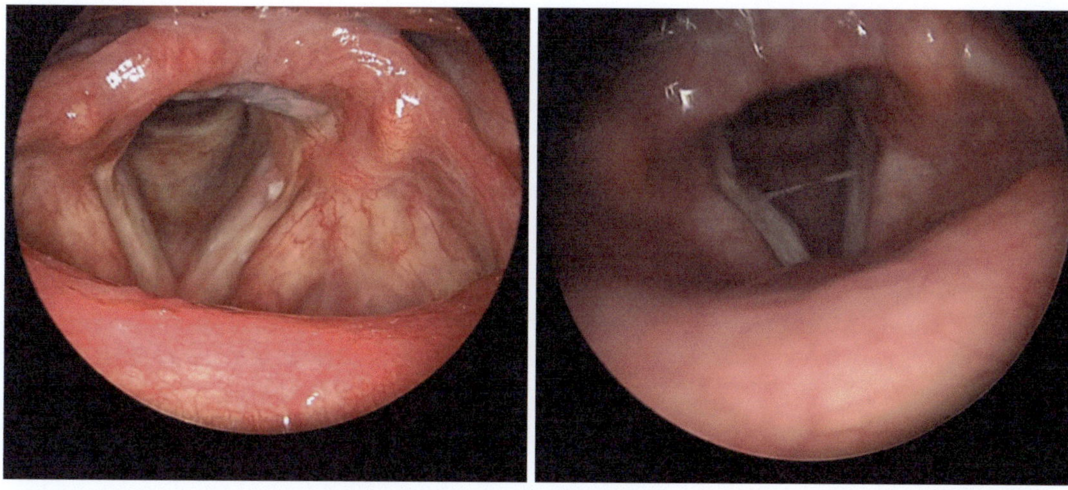

Fig. 5 Video-laryngoscopic images showing features of chronic laryngitis

without whispering. If a bacterial infection is suspected, antibiotics should be prescribed. The use of corticosteroids, although not empirically tested, is clinically beneficial in most patients with acute laryngitis.

A singer who elects to perform while the vocal folds are inflamed should be aware of the risk of permanent damage to the vocal folds and the greater risk for submucosal hemorrhage.

6. Reinke's Edema:
   It is also known as polypoid corditis. It refers to redundancy of the superficial lamina propria which appears as an outpouching of the membranous vocal folds with an edematous, almost water-balloon appearance. Based on the severity of edema, it is graded into four types.
   (i) Causes: chronic irritant exposure such as tobacco smoke, laryngopharyngeal reflux.
   (ii) Symptoms: dysphonia and sometimes dyspnea.
   (iii) Videostroboscopy: decreased mucosal wave because of the mass effect of the edema, often with phase asymmetry.
   (iv) Treatment: cessation of smoking, voice therapy, and treatment of LPR. Medical management includes steroids. Surgery is sometimes considered as an option using microflap technique.
7. Gastroesophageal Reflux Disease (GERD):
   (i) Causes: performance stress, high abdominal pressures during singing, and poor eating habits such as large meals after performances.
   (ii) Symptoms: scratchy or dry throat irritation, foreign body sensation in throat, habitual throat clearing, huskiness.
   (iii) Videostroboscopy: erythema of the arytenoid mucosa, interarytenoid pachydermia, or contact ulcers.
   (iv) Treatment: proton pump inhibitors; avoiding caffeine, alcohol, and spicy foods; eating the last meal of the day, preferably a light one, no fewer than 3 h before retiring; using bed blocks to place the bed on a mild head-to-foot slant.

6 Causes of Vocal Injuries

Vocal injuries are typically caused by a combination of factors, some of which are preventable. The most common causes include the following:

1. Performance Demands: The most frequent cause of vocal injuries is simply using the voice too much. Just like any muscle, the

vocal folds can become fatigued and damaged with excessive use, especially when the voice is not given adequate time to rest and recover.
2. Poor Technique: Singing with incorrect technique—such as straining to hit high notes, using improper breath support, or forcing the vocal folds together too tightly—can lead to injury. Lack of vocal training or guidance can exacerbate this problem. This is most commonly encountered in commercial singing, which unlike classical singing, lacks laborious training.
3. Dehydration: The vocal folds require moisture to vibrate effectively. Dehydration can cause them to become dry and stiff, increasing the risk of strain and injury.
4. Environmental Factors: Exposure to dry air, allergens, or irritants like smoke and pollution can irritate the vocal folds and lead to injury. Professionals mostly use frequent air/bus/train travel, where due to Lombard effect, they raise their voices to be heard while rehearsals (Kwok and Eslick 2017).
5. Physical and Mental Stress: Stress, whether physical (muscle tension) or mental (performance anxiety), can exacerbate poor vocal technique and contribute to muscle tension dysphonia or other injuries. Professional singers can be at a greater risk for gastroesophageal reflux disorder (GERD) through both performance stress, high abdominal pressures during singing, and poor eating habits such as large meals after performances
6. Improper Warm-Up and Cool-Down: Just as athletes need to warm up before physical activity, singers should also warm up their voices. Skipping this step or abruptly overexerting the voice can lead to vocal strain.
7. Personal Habits
   - Moderate use or abuse of alcohol causes dehydration and is detrimental to the voice.
   - Caffeine is a diuretic, and high-fat dairy products thicken mucous secretions, thereby decreasing the efficiency of vocal fold vibration.
   - Certain foods and alcohol exacerbate gastroesophageal and extraesophageal reflux.
   - Inhaled smoke is an irritant and induces esophageal reflux, which reduces vibratory efficiency. In addition, exposure to carcinogens can lead to neoplastic changes (Kwok and Eslick 2017).

7 Prevention of Vocal Injuries

Preventing vocal injuries is always preferable to treating them. Below are some strategies for maintaining vocal health:

1. Vocal exercises and proper vocal technique: Working with a trained vocal coach can help ensure that a singer is using proper breath support, posture, and vocal production. Vocal exercises promote laryngeal adjustments at the respiratory, glottic, and articulatory/resonant levels. Laryngeal muscles are trainable. Training can increase fatigue resistance, improve vocal performance, and prevent injuries associated with incorrect voice use or intense vocal demand (Oliveira et al. 2022).
2. Vocal rest and recovery: Ensuring that the voice has adequate time to rest and recover is crucial. This includes not only taking breaks during prolonged periods of singing or speaking but also ensuring periods of vocal rest between performances.
3. Hydration: Drinking plenty of water and staying hydrated is essential for maintaining the elasticity and health of the vocal folds. Avoiding dehydrating substances, such as alcohol, smoke, and caffeine, can also help.
4. Warm-up and cool-down: A good warm-up routine can prepare the vocal folds for the demands of singing, and a cool-down can help relax the voice afterward. Techniques like gentle sirens, lip trills, and humming can be effective. In the absence of dysphonia, work should be directed to vocal enhancement through the acquisition of skills, performance improvement, fatigue management, and injury prevention.
5. Avoiding vocal abuse: Common forms of voice misuse in professional voice users include (1) over-rehearsing, (2) spending too much time

working in the studio, (3) singing too loudly, and (4) singing outside the singer's capable range. In addition, commercial singing frequently incorporates artificial roughness to render "validity" to the performance.
Singers should avoid screaming, shouting, or speaking loudly for extended periods, especially if they are not accustomed to such activities. The use of microphones can help reduce vocal strain during loud performances.
6. Seeking early treatment: If any symptoms of vocal distress arise—such as hoarseness, discomfort, or vocal fatigue—it is important to seek professional help. An otolaryngologist (ENT specialist) or speech-language pathologist can help identify and treat vocal injuries early.

8 Care of Professional Voice

Professional voice users are those whose voice is vital to their line of work. Professional singers are one group of individuals that make their livelihood based entirely on their voice. Because professional singers experience tremendous vocal demands both at and outside work, they are more likely to experience voice issues themselves. Even minor voice problems can have a significant effect on these people as it jeopardizes their entire career and income. To preserve a healthy voice, it is crucial that vocalists understand the effects of excessive and improper voice use which can impact their voice. They should consider following appropriate measures by practicing vocal exercises and adhering to vocal hygiene guidelines. Maintaining a healthy voice through behaviors that keep it stable and powerful for years to come is known as vocal hygiene.

Guidelines for vocal hygiene focus on changing non-vocal behaviors that impact voice as well as vocal behaviors (Stemple et al. 2018). Non-vocal behaviors include dehydration, smoking, use of caffeine, alcohol consumption, diet, exposure to allergens, dust, and air conditioners. Vocal behaviors include throat clearing, shouting, excessive talking, and recreational voice use such as mimicry. It is important for voice users to understand the types of vocal behaviors that can harm their voice over time and work to change them.

Here are a few vocal hygiene suggestions to help keep one's voice sounding good.

- *Maintaining proper hydration*: Maintaining a healthy systemic hydration level in the body keeps mucosal tissue strong, whereas surface or superficial hydration maximizes the moisture content on the vocal folds' surface, keeping them lubricated and malleable (Weston and Schneider 2023).
- *Avoid throat clearing* too often as this can irritate it and make the vocal folds swell up. Try drinking tiny sips of water or gently swallowing if one feels the need to clear their throat. Another option is to try a mild, breathy cough that does not put as much pressure on the vocal cords.
- *Reduced caffeine intake*: While moderate caffeine intake may not directly affect the vocal folds, its diuretic effects can dehydrate the voice and cause the vocal fold mucosa to become less mobile. This can cause hoarseness and thicker phlegm, which may necessitate frequent throat clearing (Weston and Schneider 2023). However, this idea lacks strong empirical support, as the available evidence is considered inconclusive, preventing the establishment of definitive conclusions for clinical guidelines (Georgalas et al. 2023).
- *Refrain from using alcohol and smoking*: Alcohol dries up the vocal folds since it is a diuretic, just as caffeine. Limiting alcohol intake is a good idea if vocal health is important, especially before a focused voice task.
- *Smoking*: In addition to causing long-term harm like cancer, smoking also causes irritation and inflammation of the vocal cords. Giving up smoking has a major positive impact on one's general health and voice quality (Murry and Rosen 2000).
- *Environment*: Even performance environment could be quite tricky for the singers as the theatrical smoke used for enhancing the visual experience of the performance pose a negative impact on their voice. A noisy background environment leads an unknown overuse of voice to meet the task demands.

- *Profession and performance voice use*: Another concern arises for individuals who use their voice both professionally and for performance. Many singers have voice related professions, which can be very demanding. In relation to singing style (or subgenre), the worry is that, in addition to how often the voice is used, the particular type of phonation—such as variations in vocal fold closure speeds and the impact stresses resulting from different levels of adduction forces—may play a significant role in the development of vocal problems, particularly phonotrauma (Toles et al. 2022).
- *Loud speaking and shouting* can cause vocal strain and damage if one raises their voice constantly to be heard over background noise or during conversations. In order to give the voice a break during lengthy voice tasks, try to keep the speaking level reasonable and take rests.
- *Laryngopharyngeal reflux* can be prevented by extending the time between meal and bedtime. Additionally, avoiding reflux inducing eating and drinking habits can help in maintaining optimal voice (Weston and Schneider 2023).

Voice athletes, on a routine basis, must follow vocal exercise to keep the mechanism in shape. Furthermore, before an extensive vocal use, it is essential to practice vocal warm-ups to prevent stress and damage to the vocal cords (Sabol et al. 1995). This ensures clarity and improves the quality of voice. It is important to ensure that these voice athletes consult and are monitored regularly by voice pathologists or vocal coaches so that they follow the right regiments.

The following are some of the exercises that could be included:

- *Humming*: To warm up one's vocal cords, they should begin the day or any vocal sessions with mild humming. It prevents vocal hyperfunction and prepares the voice for the vocal tasks.
- *Vocal stretching*: Vocal stretches avoid strain, much like stretching one's body before working out. To keep the vocal cords flexible, practice soft glides up and down the vocal range on various musical notes according to the categories of classical singing.
- *Breathing exercises*: The health of the voice depends on proper breath support. Take a steady, deep breath through your nose, hold it for a few seconds, and then release it gradually. This encourages the use of voice in a healthy way and also reduces stress (Murry and Rosen 2000).
- *Vocal stretches*: Similar to extending your body before working out, voice stretches can help you avoid tension. Vocal cord flexibility can be preserved by practicing soft glides up and down the vocal range on various vowel sounds, such as "ah" or "ee." Slowly inhale through your nose, hold it for a short while, and then slowly exhale. In addition to encouraging appropriate voice use, this also reduces stress.
- *Lip trills and tongue trills*: Rolling the lips together and generating a sound is known as a lip trill. It enhances breath control and relaxes the voice cords, lips, and face.
  Similar to lip trills, tongue trills include rolling the tongue on the roof of the mouth. It eases the strain in the throat and the tongue.
- *Scales*: To stretch and prepare the vocal cords for use, sing scales slowly. Increase the volume gradually after starting out quietly.
- *Vocal function exercises* (Toles et al. 2022) *within and across octave can be practiced*
  Sustain vowels as long as possible on a comfortable note.
  Glide vowels from the lowest to the highest notes in the frequency range.
  Glide vowels from the highest to the lowest notes in the frequency range.
  Sustain the musical notes on the octave as long as possible.
- *Resonance*: Practice anterior focused resonance to improve vocal tract vibration and reduce laryngeal strain (Boone et al. 2005).
- *Feedback*: There are several apps available which provide feedback and assist in monitoring the pitch, loudness, and rhythm.

8.1 Lung Function in Singers, Flutists, and Nadaswaram Players

Singing can have a positive impact on lung function, particularly for individuals with respiratory conditions such as chronic obstructive pulmonary disease (COPD). The following changes are expected in singers: (i) increased lung capacity: singers tend to have greater lung capacity due to the demands of controlled breathing and sustained vocalization; (ii) improved respiratory muscle strength: singing exercises the diaphragm and other respiratory muscles, which can lead to increased strength and efficiency; (iii) enhanced breathing control: singers learn to control their breathing patterns, which can help manage lung conditions like COPD; and (iv) better gas exchange: singing may improve gas exchange by increasing dynamic lung volume and airflow, potentially benefiting individuals with respiratory diseases (Lewis et al. 2021). The physiological adaptations in singers will include (a) diaphragmatic breathing which can become a more efficient and effective way of breathing; (b) abdominal muscle activity is increased particularly in the transverse abdominis muscle, to support breathing and vocal production; and (c) control the glottic aperture to modulate airflow and support sustained vocalization. The benefits of regular singing are improved quality of life for individuals with COPD by increasing physical activity levels and enhancing respiratory muscle strength and singing can be a form of moderate physical activity that encourages individuals to engage in regular exercise and improve their overall health (Fang et al. 2022; American Lung Association n.d.).

8.2 Lung Function in Flutists

Playing the flute requires controlled breathing and can impact lung function. Flutists develop specific respiratory techniques to produce sound and sustain long phrases. The physiological adaptations in flutists include increased lung capacity, improved respiratory muscle strength, and enhanced breathing control: Flutists learn to control breathing patterns, including airflow and pressure, to produce desired tones and dynamics. The demonstrable effects on pulmonary function are increased forced expiratory volume (FEV) due to the demands of controlled exhalation, increase in forced vital capacity (FVC), and improvement in respiratory endurance: Regular flute playing can improve respiratory endurance, enabling flutists to sustain long phrases. However, overuse or poor technique can lead to respiratory fatigue or strain.

8.3 Lung Function in Nadaswaram Players

Nadaswaram is a traditional South Indian wind instrument. Studies show that nadaswaram players have (i) increased forced vital capacity (FVC): a statistically significant higher mean FVC of 2.99 L compared to other instrument players (2.11 L); (ii) improved forced expiratory volume (FEV1): a statistically significant higher mean nadaswaram players' FEV1 is 2.81 L, compared to 2.90 L for other players; and (iii) enhanced forced expiratory flow (FEF): Nadaswaram players have a higher mean FEF of 4.10 L, compared to 3.45 L for other players (Harivallavan et al. 2015).

These findings suggest that regular nadaswaram playing improves large airway function, but smaller airway function remains unaffected. The physical demands of playing the nadaswaram, a double reed wind instrument with a conical bore, likely contribute to these respiratory adaptations. As a traditional South Indian instrument, nadaswaram players develop specific breathing techniques to produce its characteristic sound, potentially enhancing their lung capacity and respiratory muscle strength (Wikipedia Contributors 2025).

9 Conclusion

Vocal injuries are a common concern for singers, as the voice is both a delicate and powerful instrument. While there are many potential causes of vocal injury, most can be mitigated through proper technique, adequate rest, and good vocal habits. By understanding the anatomy of the voice, recognizing the symptoms of injury, and taking steps to prevent strain, singers can safeguard their vocal health for a long and successful career. Preventative strategies, including regular training, hydration, and voice care, are key components of sustaining a healthy voice and minimizing the risk of injury. In the event of injury, early intervention and professional guidance are essential for a successful recovery and return to vocal performance. By taking proactive steps to care for their instrument, vocalists can continue to perform at their best, avoiding the debilitating effects of vocal injuries.

Playing the flute can have a positive impact on lung function, particularly in terms of increased lung capacity, respiratory muscle strength, and breathing control. Regular practice and proper technique are essential to maximize benefits and minimize potential risks.

Acknowledgments The authors are grateful to Dr K Sai Saranya, resident in ENT, Mazumdar Shaw Medical Centre; Adithi G. Hegde (Clinical Fellow at Narayana Health City and Dr. S. R. Chandrashekhar Institute of Speech and Hearing, Bengaluru); and Bella Mathews (Intern at Narayana Health City, Bengaluru, and Father Mullers College of Speech and Hearing, Mangaluru), for their help in preparation on the manuscript.

References

Altman KW (2007) Vocal fold masses. Otolaryngol Clin N Am 40(5):1091–1108, viii. https://doi.org/10.1016/j.otc.2007.05.011

American Lung Association (n.d.) Music therapy and lung health. Available at: https://www.lung.org/blog/music-therapy-lung-health. Accessed 20 June 2025

Arunachalam R, Boominathan P, Mahalingam S (2014) Clinical voice analysis of carnatic singers. J Voice, 28(1):128.e1–128.e9. The Voice Foundation

Boone DR, McFarlane SC, Von Berg SL, Zraick RI (2005) The voice and voice therapy, 8th edn. Pearson, Boston

Drake RL, Vogl W, Mitchell AWMK (2014) Gray's anatomy for students, 3rd edn. Elsevier, Philadelphia

Fang X, Qiao Z, Yu X, Tian R, Liu K, Han W (2022) Effect of singing on symptoms in stable COPD: a systematic review and meta-analysis. Int J Chron Obstruct Pulmon Dis 17:2893–2904. https://doi.org/10.2147/COPD.S382037

Georgalas VL, Kalantzi N, Harpur I, Kenny C (2023) The effects of caffeine on voice: a systematic review. J Voice 37(4):636.e7

Harivallavan N, Maruthainaar A, Ariyaratnam L, Sriskandaraja S, Shanmuganathan N (2015) Effect of playing Nathaswaram on lung function. Proceedings of the Annual Scientific Sessions of Faculty of Medical Sciences, University of Sri Jayewardenepura

Kwok M, Eslick GD (2017) The impact of vocal and laryngeal pathologies among professional singers: a meta-analysis. J Voice 33(1):58–65

Lewis A, Philip KEJ, Lound A et al (2021) The physiology of singing and implications for "Singing for Lung Health" as a therapy for individuals with chronic obstructive pulmonary disease. BMJ Open Respir Res 8:e000996. https://doi.org/10.1136/bmjresp-2021-000996

Murry T, Rosen CA (2000) Vocal education for the professional voice user and singer. Otolaryngol Clin N Am 33(5):967–982. https://doi.org/10.1016/s0030-6665(05)70258-9

Oliveira P, Ribeiro VV, Florencio DSF, Palhano M, Goncalves RR, Nascimento MA et al (2022) Vocal training in healthy individuals: a scoping review. J Voice 38(5):1250.e11–1250.e23

Sabol JW, Lee L, Stemple JC (1995) The value of vocal function exercises in the practice regimen of singers. J Voice 9(1):27–36. https://doi.org/10.1016/s0892-1997(05)80220-6

Stemple JC, Roy N, Klaben BK (2018) Clinical voice pathology: theory and management, 5th edn. Plural Publishing, San Diego

Toles LE, Ortiz AJ, Marks KL, Mehta DD, Van Stan JH, Hillman RE (2022) Amount and characteristics of speaking and singing voice use in vocally healthy female college student singers during a typical week. J Voice 36(2):203–211. https://doi.org/10.1016/j.jvoice.2020.04.029

Wang X, Jiang W, Zheng X, Xue Q (2021) A computational study of the effects of vocal fold stiffness parameters on voice production. J Acoust Soc Am. https://doi.org/10.1016/j.jvoice.2019.09.004

Weston Z, Schneider SL (2023) Demystifying vocal hygiene: considerations for professional voice users. Curr Otorhinolaryngol Rep 11:387–394. https://doi.org/10.1007/s40136-023-00494-x

Wikipedia Contributors (2025) Nadaswaram. Wikipedia. Available at: https://en.wikipedia.org/w/index.php?title=Nadaswaram&oldid=1286803175. Accessed 20 June 2025

Injuries Specific to Instrumental Music and Radiological Features: Non-percussion Instruments

Kanaka Durga Prasad Bhamidipaty,
Rajesh Botchu, and Veenadhari Bhamidipaty

Contents

K. D. P. Bhamidipaty
Department of Radiodiagnosis, NRIIMS, Visakhapatnam, India

R. Botchu
Department of MSK Radiology, Royal Orthopaedic Hospital, Birmingham, UK

V. Bhamidipaty (✉)
Department of CSE, GITAM, Visakhapatnam, India

Med Radiol Diagn Imaging (2025)
https://doi.org/10.1007/174_2025_638,
Published Online: 31 October 2025

Abstract

Non-percussion musicians—those who play string, wind, and keyboard instruments—are frequently exposed to physical demands that may lead to musculoskeletal injuries. Unlike percussionists, whose injuries often stem from impact and vibration, non-percussionists are at risk due to repetitive motions, awkward postures, prolonged static positions, and asymmetrical use of the body. These conditions are often exacerbated by inadequate ergonomics, intense practice schedules, and performance anxiety. This chapter explores the various types of injuries associated with playing non-percussion instruments, highlighting their causes, manifestations, and management. Drawing on clinical studies, musician testimonies, and ergonomic principles, this chapter also discusses preventive strategies and rehabilitation techniques tailored for the musical population.

1 Introduction

Playing a musical instrument demands precision, control, and endurance—qualities that are not only mentally taxing but physically strenuous. Non-percussion musicians, such as violinists, flautists, pianists, and saxophonists, often spend long hours in practice and performance, adopting postures that are ergonomically challenging. As a result, many suffer from a variety of injuries that can range from mild discomfort to debilitating chronic pain.

Performance-related musculoskeletal disorders (PRMDs) are particularly prevalent among musicians, with some studies estimating their incidence at over 80% in professional instrumentalists (Zaza 1998). This chapter aims to explore the nature and causes of injuries in musicians who play non-percussion instruments, focusing on biomechanics, playing techniques, and occupational stressors. It also examines preventive approaches, treatment modalities, and the role of education in reducing injury risk.

2 Epidemiology of Injuries in Non-percussion Musicians

Research consistently shows that musicians are a high-risk group for work-related injuries. Violinists and violists, for instance, commonly report shoulder, neck, and back pain due to the elevated arm position required during playing (Brandfonbrener 2009). Wind instrumentalists often suffer from facial pain, jaw problems, and respiratory strain, while pianists are prone to repetitive strain injuries (RSIs) affecting the wrists and forearms.

The prevalence of PRMDs among musicians varies by instrument, age, and level of professionalism. According to a large survey conducted by Ackermann et al. (2012), string players had the highest injury rates, followed by keyboard and woodwind players. Female musicians reported more complaints than males, possibly due to anatomical and ergonomic differences.

3 Biomechanical and Ergonomic Stressors

3.1 String Instruments

String instrument players, such as violinists, violists, cellists, and guitarists, often experience asymmetrical loading of the upper body. The left shoulder and neck support the instrument, while the left hand performs intricate finger movements. The right hand, meanwhile, handles bowing or plucking motions. This uneven posture leads to muscle imbalances and joint strain, particularly in the trapezius, deltoid, and rotator cuff muscles (Watson 2009).

3.2 Keyboard Instruments

Pianists and organists face challenges due to prolonged sitting, static arm positions, and continuous wrist extension and flexion. Overuse of the wrist extensors and flexors, especially in high-speed or loud passages, often results in tendinitis or tenosynovitis. Poor posture, non-adjustable benches, and incorrect keyboard height further contribute to discomfort and injury (Fry 1986).

3.3 Wind Instruments

Woodwind and brass players may develop overuse injuries in facial, cervical, and thoracic regions. Holding heavy instruments like the saxophone can strain the neck and shoulders. The embouchure—the positioning of facial muscles and lips on the mouthpiece—requires fine motor control and sustained contraction, potentially leading to orofacial pain, temporomandibular joint dysfunction (TMJD), and even dental issues (Rickert et al. 2013).

4 Common Injuries in Non-percussion Instrumentalists

4.1 Repetitive Strain Injury (RSI)

RSI refers to a group of conditions caused by repetitive movement, forceful exertion, and poor posture. It includes tendinitis, carpal tunnel syndrome, bursitis (Fig. 1), and De Quervain's tenosynovitis (Figs. 2 and 3). Pianists and violinists are particularly susceptible due to rapid finger movements and sustained arm positions (Fry 1986).

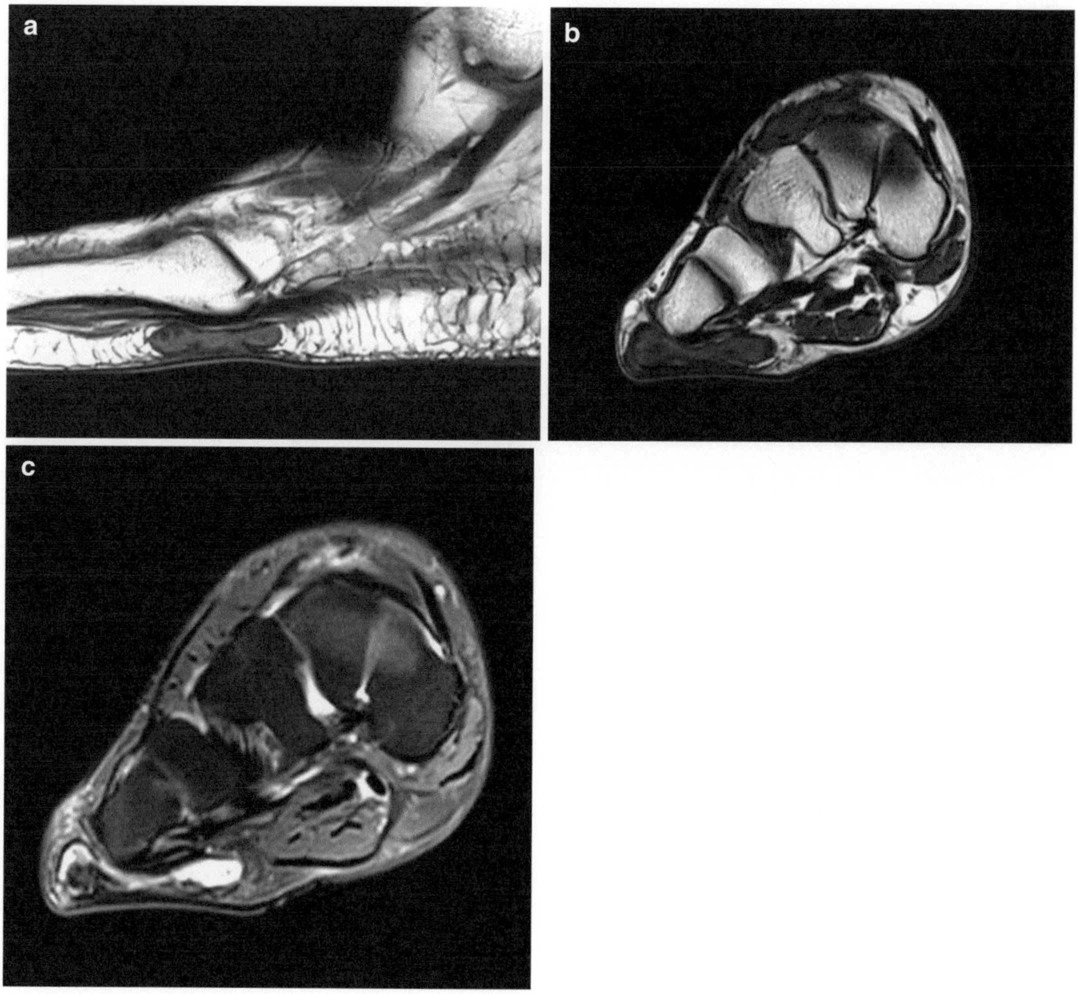

Fig. 1 Sagittal PD (**a**), coronal PD (**b**), and PDFS (**c**) [MRI] showing adventitious bursitis in relation the plantar aspect of the base of 5th metatarsal. (Source: Author)

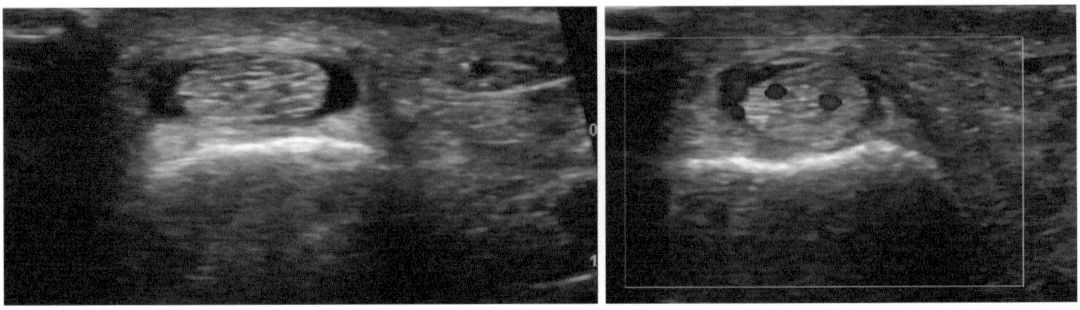

Fig. 2 Short axis ultrasound showing moderate tenosynovitis of extensor capri ulnaris with mild increased signal on Doppler. (Source: Author)

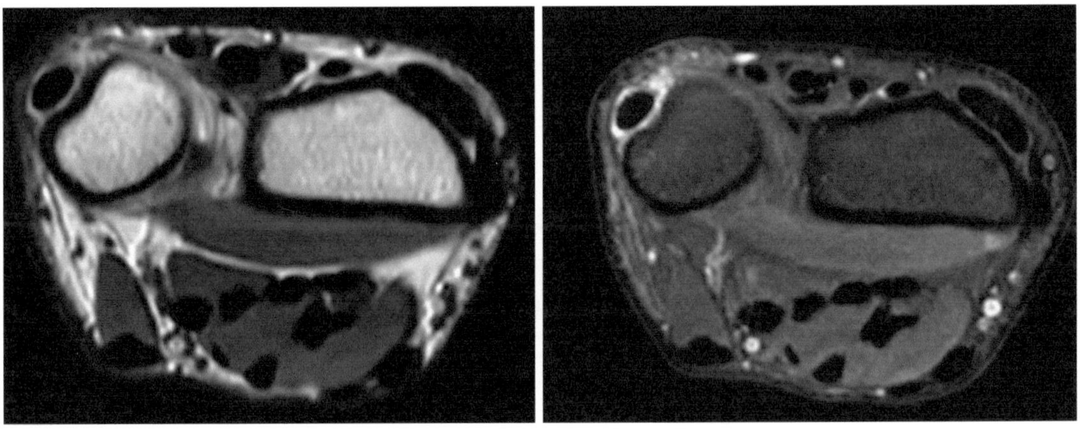

Fig. 3 PD and PDFS (MRI) axial showing marked tenosynovitis of extensor carpi ulnaris. (Source: Author)

4.2 Thoracic Outlet Syndrome (TOS)

This condition involves compression of the brachial plexus or blood vessels between the neck and the shoulder. Violinists and violists, who often elevate and rotate their shoulders, are at risk. Symptoms include numbness, tingling, and weakness in the arm (Brandfonbrener 2009).

4.3 Focal Dystonia

Focal dystonia is a neurological condition in which involuntary muscle contractions interfere with motor control. It often affects keyboard players and string musicians, manifesting as finger curling or loss of coordination. Though rare, it can be career-ending without proper management (Altenmüller and Jabusch 2010).

4.4 Temporomandibular Joint Dysfunction (TMJD) (Figs. 4, 5, and 6)

Wind instrumentalists who maintain prolonged jaw tension may develop TMJD. This presents as jaw pain, clicking sounds, or difficulty chewing. Clarinettists and oboists who use a tight embouchure are particularly prone (Rickert et al. 2013).

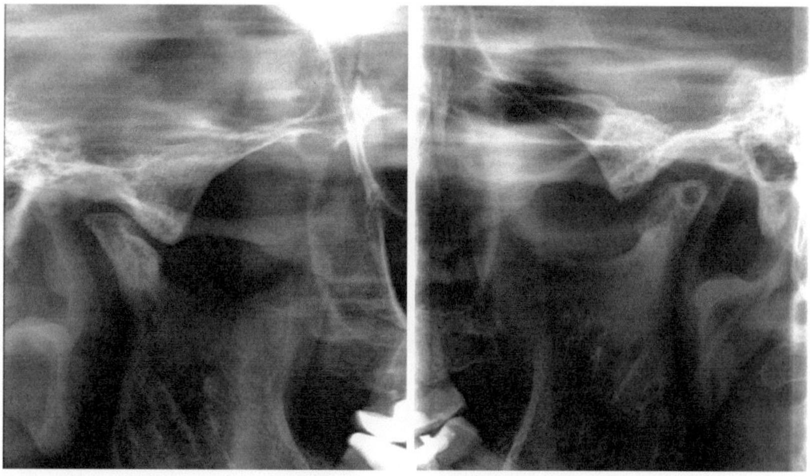

Fig. 4 Radiograph showing marked degenerative of temporomandibular joint. (Source: Author)

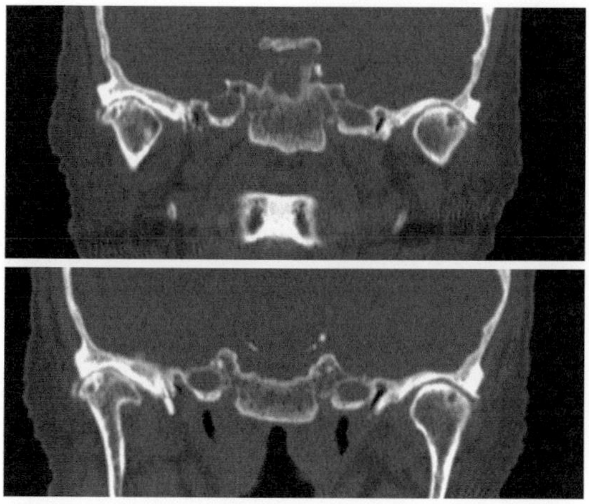

Fig. 5 Coronal CT showing marked degenerative of both temporomandibular joints. (Source: Author)

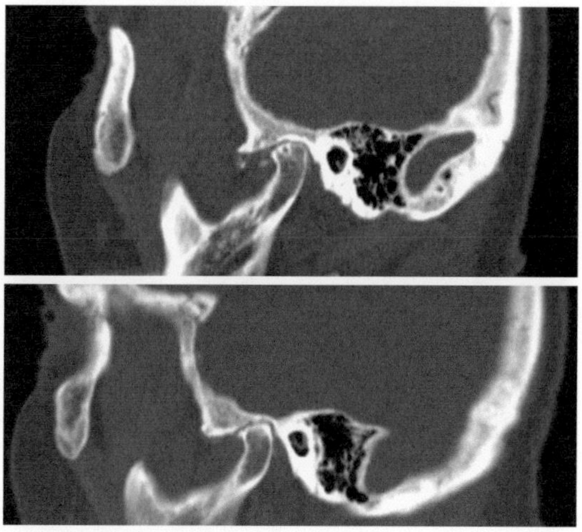

Fig. 6 Sagittal CT showing marked degenerative of temporomandibular joint. (Source: Author)

4.5 Back (Fig. 7) and Neck Pain (Fig. 8)

Musicians who sit or stand for long durations without adequate support often suffer from back and neck pain. Poorly designed chairs or music stands, improper playing posture, and insufficient breaks all contribute to spinal stress, especially in cellists and keyboard players (Zaza 1998).

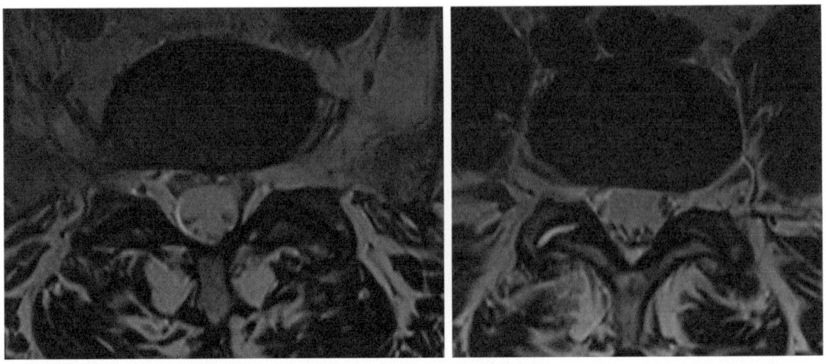

Fig. 7 Axial T2 showing moderate facet joint degeneration at L4/L5. (Source: Author)

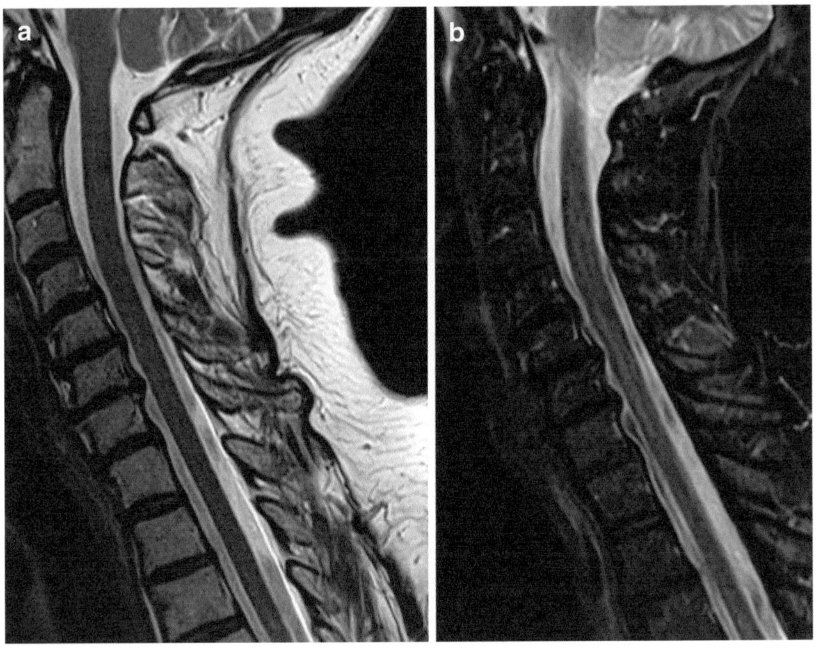

Fig. 8 Sagittal T1 (**a**) and STIR (**b**) showing small disc bulges and disc dehydration at multiple levels in keeping with degenerative change. (Source: Author)

5 Instrument-Specific Skin and Tissue Conditions

In addition to musculoskeletal injuries, non-percussion instrumentalists often experience dermatological and superficial tissue problems resulting from prolonged and repetitive contact with their instruments. These conditions, though often overlooked, can cause significant discomfort and impact performance quality.

5.1 Violinist's Neck

A well-documented condition, *violinist's neck* refers to localized irritation, lichenification, and pigmentation changes that occur on the left side of the neck and jawline, where the violin or viola is typically supported. This condition is caused by chronic pressure, friction from the instrument, and accumulation of sweat and rosin dust. It may present as erythema, eczema-like patches, or darkened thickened skin, particularly in players who do not

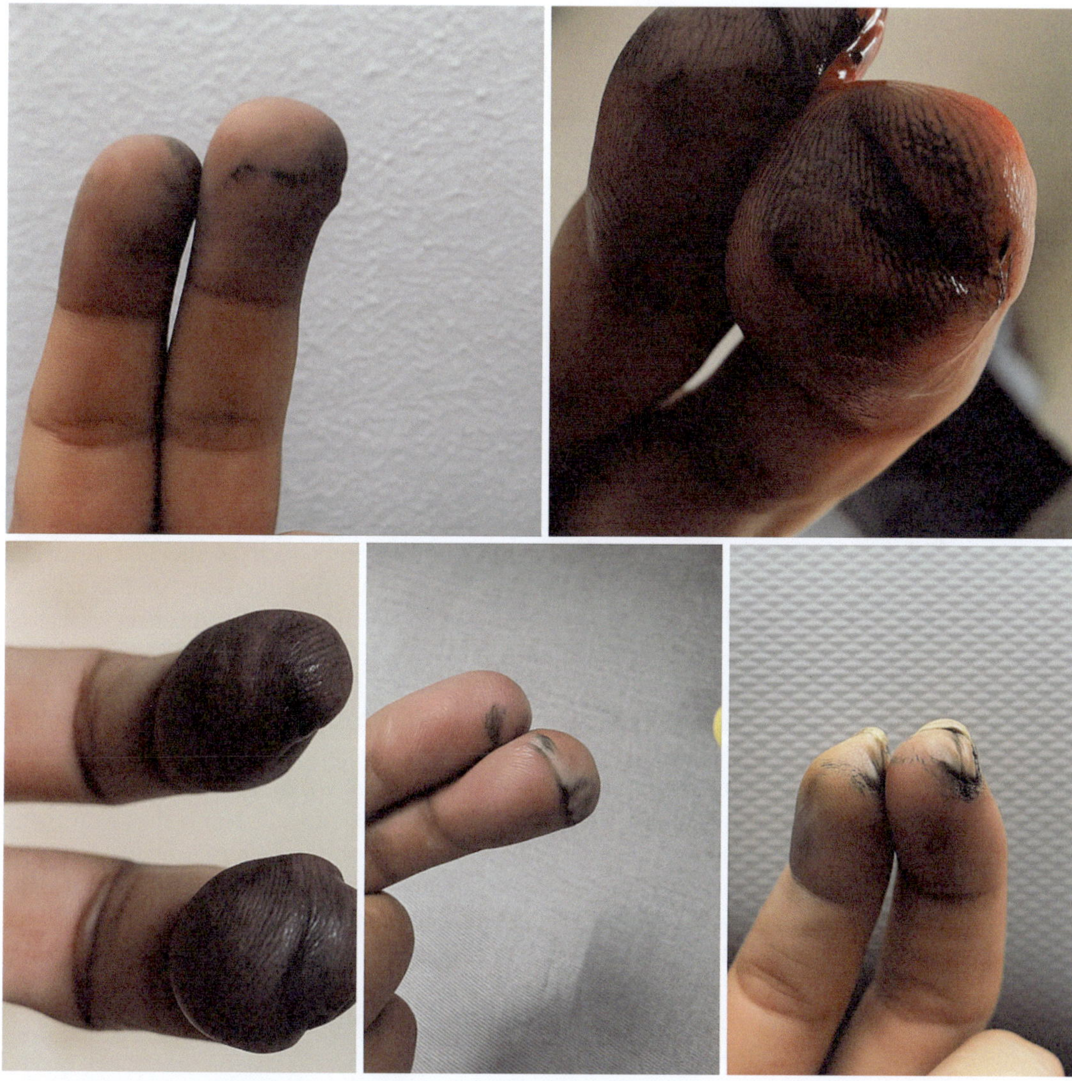

Fig. 9 Vainikas fingers in different artists of veena instrument. (Source: Author)

use chin or shoulder rests (Gupta and Gupta 2011). While primarily a cosmetic and discomfort-related issue, violinist's neck can lead to secondary infections or increased sensitivity in some cases.

5.2 Vainikas Fingers (Fig. 9)

In Indian string players, especially those playing the *veena* or *sitar*, a unique condition called *Vainikas fingers* which is being described for the first time. This involves hypertrophy and stiffness of the fingertips, along with deep grooves and keratin buildup on the distal phalanges of the left hand. The condition arises from constant contact with steel or brass strings, and though often painless, it can occasionally impair tactile sensitivity and fine control, particularly during long recitals or practice sessions.

5.3 Hyperkeratosis, Callosities, and Fissures

Frequent mechanical stress on the fingertips, palms, or other areas of skin can lead to hyperkeratosis—an abnormal thickening of the outer skin layer. This is commonly seen in guitarists, cellists, and veena players who use their fingers for plucking or pressing strings. Over time, this protective response leads to callosities—hardened, raised patches of skin that reduce pain but may alter finger sensitivity. In some cases, particularly during dry weather or excessive practice, fissures or cracks may develop, which are painful and can lead to bleeding or infections (Brandfonbrener 2009).

5.4 Scaling and Dermatitis

Players of woodwind and brass instruments, especially those in prolonged physical contact with metal parts, may experience scaling, dryness, or allergic contact dermatitis. These conditions can affect the lips, fingers, or areas where the instrument is gripped or pressed against the skin. Poor hygiene, perspiration, and lack of protective padding contribute to these skin changes.

Though these conditions are typically not as severe as musculoskeletal disorders, they can interfere with practice, lead to pain or cosmetic concerns, and reduce performance efficiency. Preventive measures include using protective tapes or pads, maintaining instrument hygiene, moisturizing affected skin areas, and modifying technique or playing posture as needed.

6 Psychological and Environmental Factors

Musicians often experience high levels of psychological stress due to performance pressure, competition, and perfectionism. This mental strain can exacerbate physical symptoms or delay recovery. Inadequate sleep, poor nutrition, and lack of physical conditioning further reduce resilience to injury (Kenny and Ackermann 2015).

Moreover, the environment in which a musician practices or performs plays a critical role. Factors such as lighting, room temperature, acoustics, and equipment design can all influence posture and technique. Poor ergonomics during long rehearsals or gigs increase the risk of chronic injuries.

7 Prevention Strategies

7.1 Ergonomic Adjustments

Adjusting the musician's environment can drastically reduce injury risk. Examples include using adjustable benches, music stands at eye level, and instrument supports such as shoulder rests and chin pads for violinists. For keyboard players, correct seat height and wrist alignment are critical.

7.2 Warm-Up and Stretching

Just as athletes warm up before competition, musicians should prepare their bodies with gentle stretches and mobility exercises. Dynamic warm-ups targeting the wrists, shoulders, and back can enhance blood flow and flexibility.

7.3 Technique and Training

Proper instruction in technique is vital. For instance, keyboard players should avoid excessive finger lifting, and string players should use relaxed bow holds. Regular feedback from experienced teachers or physiotherapists can help detect poor habits early.

7.4 Scheduled Breaks and Pacing

Musicians should adopt practice routines that include short, frequent breaks to allow muscle recovery. Techniques such as the Pomodoro method (25 min of focused work followed by a 5-min break) can help maintain focus without fatigue.

7.5 Physical Conditioning

Cross-training with aerobic and strength exercises improves general fitness and injury resistance. Core strengthening is especially beneficial for postural support in sitting or standing musicians (Zaza 1998).

8 Treatment and Rehabilitation

The management of musician injuries requires a multidisciplinary approach. Treatment may involve the following:

Physiotherapy: Includes manual therapy, ultrasound, and neuromuscular re-education to restore function.

Occupational Therapy: Focuses on adapting tools and environments to the musician's needs.

Medication: Anti-inflammatory drugs or muscle relaxants may be used temporarily under supervision.

Psychological Support: Cognitive-behavioral therapy (CBT) can help manage performance anxiety and the psychological impact of injury.

Retraining and Gradual Return to Playing: A phased return plan helps rebuild endurance and confidence while minimizing the chance of reinjury.

Early intervention is crucial. Delayed treatment can lead to chronic pain, compensatory issues, or in severe cases, the end of a musical career.

9 Education and Advocacy

Musicians often lack awareness of injury risks and preventive strategies. Educational programs—especially in conservatories and music schools—should integrate topics such as musician health, body mechanics, and wellness. Teachers and institutions have a responsibility to foster a culture that values rest, technique, and self-care over relentless practice.

Professional bodies and unions can advocate for better working conditions, accessible healthcare, and research funding to support musician health.

10 Conclusion

Non-percussion musicians dedicate their lives to perfecting their art, often at great physical cost. The nature of their instruments, combined with intense practice and performance schedules, puts them at risk for a wide range of injuries. Understanding the biomechanical, psychological, and environmental factors that contribute to these conditions is essential for prevention and treatment.

With appropriate ergonomic practices, physical conditioning, and education, many injuries can be avoided or effectively managed. A holistic approach—one that respects the musician's artistry while prioritizing their health—can ensure that their passion for music continues without compromising their physical well-being.

References

Ackermann B, Adams R, Marshall E (2012) Playing-related musculoskeletal pain in upper strings players: a systematic review. Med Probl Perform Art 27(4):193–200

Altenmüller E, Jabusch HC (2010) Focal dystonia in musicians: phenomenology, pathophysiology, triggering factors, and treatment. Med Probl Perform Art 25(1):3–9

Brandfonbrener AG (2009) Musculoskeletal problems of instrumental musicians. Hand Clin 19(2):231–239

Fry HJH (1986) Overuse syndrome in musicians: prevention and management. Lancet 328(8509):728–731

Gupta L, Gupta R (2011) Violinist's neck: a classical case of frictional dermatitis. Indian J Dermatol 56(6):717–718

Kenny DT, Ackermann B (2015) Performance-related musculoskeletal pain, depression and music performance anxiety in professional orchestral musicians: a population study. Psychol Music 43(1):43–60

Rickert DL, Barrett MS, Ackermann BJ (2013) Injury and the orchestral environment: part I. Med Probl Perform Art 28(2):65–72

Watson AHD (2009) The biology of musical performance and performance-related injury. Scarecrow Press, Plymouth

Zaza C (1998) Playing-related musculoskeletal disorders in musicians: a systematic review of incidence and prevalence. Can Med Assoc J 158(8):1019–1025

Injuries Specific to Instrumental Music and Radiological Features: Percussion Instruments

Kanaka Durga Prasad Bhamidipaty, Rajesh Botchu, and Veenadhari Bhamidipaty

Contents

K. D. P. Bhamidipaty
Department of Radiodiagnosis, NRIIMS, Visakhapatnam, India

R. Botchu
Department of MSK Radiology, Royal Orthopaedic Hospital, Birmingham, UK

V. Bhamidipaty (✉)
Department of CSE, GITAM, Visakhapatnam, India

Med Radiol Diagn Imaging (2025)
https://doi.org/10.1007/174_2025_633,
Published Online: 11 November 2025

Abstract

Percussionists bring rhythm and intensity to music—but behind the energetic beats and dynamic movements lies a unique set of physical challenges. Unlike other instrumentalists, percussionists often engage the entire body in their performance, relying heavily on repetitive striking motions, forceful arm movements, and full-body coordination. These demands place them at risk for a range of musculoskeletal and overuse injuries, particularly in the hands, wrists, shoulders, and spine. This chapter explores the spectrum of performance-related injuries encountered by percussion musicians, from acute trauma to chronic overuse syndromes. It examines the role of technique, posture, instrument design, and practice habits in injury development, and offers evidence-based strategies for prevention, treatment, and rehabilitation. With insights drawn from clinical research and real-world musician experiences, this chapter aims to bridge the gap between rhythm and wellness—ensuring that percussionists can continue to perform without compromising their physical health.

1 Introduction

Overuse injuries (e.g., tendinitis, carpal tunnel syndrome), acute injuries (e.g., sprains, fractures), nerve compression syndromes (e.g., ulnar nerve entrapment), and auditory issues (e.g., hearing loss due to prolonged exposure to loud sounds) are common among percussionists (Workman 2013; May 1994).

This research will focus mostly on the different injuries and issues faced by Mridangam, Thavil, Ghatam, Kanjira, Morsing, and Tabla students and artists. Playing the mridangam involves repetition of hand movements, postures, and striking techniques, which can result in acute and chronic musculoskeletal injuries (McKinney 2010; Workman 1999).

2 Finger and Palm Injuries

I. *Skin Blisters*:

(a) Repeated striking of the fingers on the drumhead can lead to friction burns, blisters, or hardened skin on the finger's phalanx and palm (Molina 2018).

(b) In the case of a Mridangam and Tabla plater, the upper part of the palm, where the fingers begin, often comes into repeated contact with the edge of the drumhead, known as the *Boddu/Gajra*—a braided rim made of buffalo skin. This repeated striking can lead to hardened skin or discomfort over time. Over time, these blisters harden and develop into permanent calluses on the palm

(c) Another common issue among Mridangam, Ghatam, and Tabla players is the development of blisters on the index finger. This is primarily due to the frequent use of the syllable *Nam/Na*, where the index finger repeatedly strikes the treble drumhead.

(d) Another blister can be seen on the middle finger and ring finger on the dominant hand of some Mridangam and Tabla artists because the finger is constantly rubbing on the middle black patch of the treble drumhead, known as the *Karanai/Karana* for Mridangam, and *Syahi* for Tabla

(e) Moreover, the Thavil player uses caps and rings to strike the treble drumhead of the instrument. Due to constant impact, blisters develop on the fingertips over time.

(f) Blisters on the phalanx of the fingers are very common for Ghatam artists. Since the Ghatam is made of solid clay, the constant striking of fingers against its hard surface can lead to the formation of blisters and the gradual hardening of the skin. One of the most common areas affected is the edge of the distal phalanx of the thumbs, as both thumbs are frequently used to strike the instrument.

(g) Compared to Mridangam, Tabla, and Ghatam players, the Kanjira artists experience fewer blisters. However, blisters are commonly found on the phalanx of the index finger. Additionally, the edge of the palm may harden due to the rapid hand movements, leading to friction burns.

II. *Skin Abrasion*:

(a) Skin abrasions on the wrist crease, particularly near the edge of the palm, are commonly observed in some Mridangam, Thavil, and Tabla players. These abrasions occur due to the repetitive rubbing and rolling of the wrist against the bass drumhead while performing the *Gumki* (Mridangam/Thavil) *Ge* (Tabla), a technique used to produce bass modulation effects sound.

(b) Further, since the Thavil player wears caps around their fingers to strike the drumhead, the constant impact can cause pain and tear the fingertips. Additionally, abrasions may develop when a blister breaks inside the cap due to continuous striking on the drumhead.

(c) For a Ghatam player, as the skin hardens and blisters begin to form, continuous striking on the same spot leads to abrasions on the fingertips. Over time, these blisters can break, causing the skin to tear while playing.

(d) In the case of a Kanjira player, as mentioned above, some artists rest their thumb on the outer rim of the frame while holding the Kanjira. This can cause abrasions on the side of the proximal phalanx of the thumb due to repeated contact and pressure.

(e) Additionally, for a Morsing player, the plucking reed which he/she plucked repeated, is also known as the "Blade." Continuous plucking can cause abrasion on the tip of the index or middle finger.

III. *Bruises and Swelling*:

(a) Intense practice sessions can cause swelling and bruises (Workman 2003), especially on the fingertips of both hands for most of the percussionists. For certain strokes, such as *Gumki/Ge*, the player rubs their lower palm against the surface of the bass head, which can cause bruises on the lower part of the palm/wrist crease, especially for Mridangam, Thavil, and Tabla players.

(b) Additionally, for a Thavil player continuously holding and striking with the stick can lead to swelling in the palm, as the player must grip the stick tightly for extended periods.

(c) For a Ghatam player, the lower palm of the left hand (near the wrist crease) is frequently used to strike the Ghatam, in an up-and-down motion, which can result in bruising on the wrist crease. Over time, these bruises may develop into abrasions. Additionally, since the entire palm of the left hand is often used to strike the mouth of the Ghatam, repeated impact can lead to swelling in the palm.

(d) In the case of a Kanjira artist, the non-dominant hand grips the frame tightly, which may lead to swelling in the palm. Further, the tips of the fingers pressing against the drumhead experience constant pressure, sometimes resulting in bruising.

3 Tendon and Muscle Strain

I. *Tendinitis*:

(a) Overuse of tendons in the shoulders and elbows can result in inflammation, leading to joint pain and stiffness, for almost all the percussionists.

(b) The most common injuries among Mridangam, Thavil, Kanjira, and Tabla players include inflammation of the tendons in the wrists, elbows, and shoulders, leading to joint pain and stiffness (Workman 1999).

(c) For a Ghatam and Morsing player, inflammation of the tendons in the elbow is common, as the elbow is continuously tucked while playing the instrument.

(d) Regarding a Morsing player, the dominant hand's wrist undergoes continuous radial and ulnar deviation movements, which may lead to tendon pain.

II. *Muscle Pain*:

(a) For Mridangam players, angling the arm at a certain angle while practicing can lead to muscle pains (McKinney 2010) in the deltoid of the shoulder, biceps brachii, brachialis of the upper arm, and extensor carpi muscles of the forearm.

(b) Thavil players often experience muscle pain in the deltoid of the shoulders, the biceps brachii and triceps brachii of the upper arm, and the extensor carpi radialis brevis in the forearm.

(c) In the matter of a Ghatam player, muscle pain commonly occurs in the deltoid and biceps brachii muscles of the upper arm, as well as in the triceps brachii, brachioradialis, and extensor carpi radialis longus muscles of the forearm.

(d) Regarding a Kanjira player, since the forearm remains perpendicular to the upper arm while playing, tension builds up in muscles such as the deltoid, biceps brachii, brachialis, brachioradialis, and extensor carpi radialis longus. This prolonged strain can cause muscle discomfort and fatigue. Additionally, because the Kanjira is played using only one hand, the dominant hand experiences greater stiffness and strain, while the non-dominant hand remains relatively underused, potentially leading to muscular imbalance.

(e) In the case of a Morsing player, tucking the elbow and holding the instrument near the mouth can lead to muscle pain in the brachialis and biceps brachii of the upper arm, as well as the extensor carpi radialis longus in the forearm. Additionally, prolonged sitting in a cross-legged position may cause muscle pain in the thighs and calves.

(f) For a Tabla player, muscle pain may develop in the deltoid muscle of the shoulders; biceps brachii, brachioradialis, extensor carpi radialis longus muscles of the upper arm; and in the extensor carpi radialis longus of the forearm due to continuous playing.

(g) Prolonged sitting in a cross-legged posture, for almost all the percussionists, can also cause muscle pain in the upper thigh muscles area due to sustained pressure of the instrument in some cases and reduced blood circulation.

4 Joint Problems

I. *Shoulder, Elbow, and Wrist Strain*:

(a) Poor posture or techniques can lead to strain on the shoulder, elbow, and wrist joints over time, due to repetitive motion and sustained impact for almost all percussionists (Haas 2003).

II. *Thumb Joints*:

(a) In the case of a Kanjira player especially, the interphalangeal (IP) joint and metacarpophalangeal (MCP) joint of the thumb in the non-dominant hand may experience pain, particularly in players who bend their thumb inward and place it inside the frame of the Kanjira while holding it.

5 Backache and Neck Pain

I. *Back Pain*:

(a) Sitting and leaning the torso excessively toward the instrument, or tending to slouch/bend the back while playing for extended periods, can lead to strain and stiffness on the spine, resulting in back pain faced by almost all the percussionists (Paris 1995).

(b) Moreover, regarding a Thavil player, since the Thavil is played in a standing position during processions, carrying the heavy instrument can strain the spine. Moreover, players often need to walk while playing, which can lead to pain in the lower back and hips.

(c) Furthermore, prolonged sitting in a cross-legged posture may cause lower back pain, particularly due to the stress placed on the lower spine, for almost all percussionists.

II. *Neck Pain*:

(a) Bending the neck forward while practicing can lead to axial neck pain which is very often an injury among Mridangam, Thavil, Morsing, and Tabla artists.

(b) While standing and playing, some Thavil players habitually bend their necks forward, which can lead to axial neck pain as mentioned above. This can result in the player's neck and back being hunched over time.

(c) Moreover, while playing the Morsing, players often develop the habit of pushing their neck forward, which is very common and can lead to axial neck pain.

6 Leg Issues

I. *Cramp*:

(a) In the case of some players, such as Mridangam, Thavil, and Ghatam players, while placing the instrument on the leg or the laps for a long period, the calf muscles on the leg (for Mridangam and Thavil), or the thighs can suddenly tighten and cause cramps. These cramps (Molina 2018) can cause pain to the calf muscles, thigh muscles, and feet of these performers.

(b) Moreover, sitting cross-legged for an extended period can cause discomfort and muscle cramps in the thighs due to reduced blood circulation and prolonged muscle tension, for almost all the percussionists mentioned above.

II. *Edema*:

(a) Sitting for long periods with the weight of the instrument pressing on the feet (in the case of Mridangam and Thavil players), or simply sitting down cross-legged, can cause the ankles to swell, darken, and bulge, a condition known as "edema." This happens because gravity pulls fluid down into the lower legs and ankles, and it is very common among all percussionists.

7 Mental Injuries (Especially in the Case of a Kanjira Player)

I. *Mental Fatigue*: Since Kanjira players must reproduce complex rhythmic patterns (Mridangam players execute with both hands) using only one hand, they require heightened focus and concentration. This continuous mental effort can lead to fatigue over time (Harnsberger 2008).

II. Morsing artists also experience mental fatigue due to the requirement to coordinate breathing, plucking, and vocal modulation (Paris 1995).

8 Mouth Issues (Especially in the Matter of a Morsing Player)

I. *Tooth Pain/Damage*: Holding the Morsing (made of metal) between the front teeth can lead to corrosion due to interaction with saliva, potentially causing tooth sensitivity (Workman 2013).

II. *Jaw Strain*: Placing the Morsing between the teeth can lead to temporomandibular joint (TMJ) disorder. Clenching the instrument too tightly inside the mouth may cause jaw discomfort.

III. *Lip Injury*: Plucking the reed, which extends out of the mouth, can cause bruises, small tears, and bleeding on the lips.

IV. *Tongue Injury*: While playing, it is advised to keep the tongue rolled inside the mouth. If it comes into contact with the central steel rod, it may cause injuries such as tears and bleeding.

V. *Gum Injury*: Holding the instrument against the teeth can cause gum soreness and minor bleeding due to excessive pressure.

9 Breathing and Throat Issues (Mostly Regarding a Morsing Player)

I. *Overbreathing or Dizziness*: If the player breathes too fast, fatigue may increase, leading to shortness of breath and dizziness.

II. *Throat Irritation*: Excessive vocalization or throat control can lead to throat discomfort.

10 Factors Contributing to Injuries: Instrument-Specific Risk Factors (e.g., Drumsticks, Mallets, Keyboard Percussion), Repetitive Strain due to Prolonged Practice Sessions, Poor Posture or Improper Technique, Impact of Environmental Factors (e.g., Stage Setup, Lighting, Temperature)

Several factors contribute to injuries among Mridangam, Thavil, Ghatam, Kanjira, Morsing, and Tabla students and artists, varying from physical demands to improper techniques. This study focuses mostly on the factors contributing to injuries for all the percussionists mentioned above regarding the injuries mentioned above. Some of the factors are as follows.

10.1 Instrument-Specific Risk Factors

A. In the Case of a Mridangam Player: *Drumhead Materials*:

I. The materials used to make the drumheads are a significant factor contributing to the blisters that Mridangam players often develop on their fingers. A specific type of Mridangam, known as the *Kappi Mridangam*, features a treble drumhead made of buffalo skin rather than the more commonly used cow or goat skin by certain Mridangam players. Buffalo skin is relatively thicker, requiring greater effort and force to strike the drumhead effectively. Repeatedly striking with excessive force can lead to blisters on the fingers (Workman 1999). This is one reason why many Mridangam players can be seen wearing white finger bandages on their index fingers for protection.

Another factor contributing to finger blisters is the black patch at the center of the treble drumhead, known as the *Karanai* or *Karana*, on the Mridangam. Continuous striking and rapid rubbing on this black patch during playing can cause blisters, particularly on the index and middle fingers.

The continuous striking of those blisters on the finger can lead to the breaking of those blisters, which can result in a literal cut on the finger, which can be very painful.

II. Another risk factor for injuries in Mridangam players is bruising on the wrist caused by playing the bass drumhead, known as the *Thoppi*. The structure of the *Thoppi* consists of two outer layers of buffalo skin arranged as concentric rings and an inner layer made of goat skin. When these three layers are tied together, a noticeable gap forms between the outer buffalo skin and the inner goat skin. It is important to note that the bass drumhead is not a flat surface; the outer buffalo skin is slightly elevated compared to the inner goat skin, creating this gap.

While performing the *Gumki* technique, the player must roll or slide the edge of their palm inside the inner layer, striking the goat skin with the fingertips. This repeated motion causes the wrist to rub against the edge of the raised buffalo skin, which can result in bruising over time.

Ergonomics of the Instrument

I. The weight of the Mridangam is one of the risk factors that contribute to injuries such as cramps, edema of the ankle, and fractures. We must note that the shell of the Mridangam is made of wood, which can weigh between 7 and 16 kg approximately, depending on the height and type of wood the instrument is made of.
Hence, placing the Mridangam on the calf muscle of the leg for a prolonged time can result in the cramping of the calf muscles and feet of the student/artist.
Too much heavy pressure of the instrument weight can cause the ankle to swell and become black and bulged. Continuous pressure on the ankle can cause a phenomenon called "Edema," causing swelling in the ankle led by a build-up of fluid in the body's tissues. This swollen ankle will cause discomfort to the performer while sitting down and practicing.
Fractures of the leg bones, such as the tibia or fibula, are rare, but these can occur due to the weight of the Mridangam. This risk is especially high among young learners, whose bones are still developing and more fragile. If the Mridangam accidentally falls on a child's leg while they are attempting to position it in the desired posture, it can result in a fracture.

II. Another rare injury in this category is back and neck pain, historically associated with traditional practices. In earlier times, groups would perform *Sankeerthana* during God's processions on the streets, where players would tie the Mridangam around their neck and shoulders using a cloth. The weight of the instrument, combined with prolonged carrying and playing, often led to strain, resulting in neck and back pain, hence making the Mridangam artist slightly hunched over time.

B. In the Case of a Thavil Player: *Thavil Kattai Practice*

I. When learning the Thavil, a student begins by practicing on a wooden frame known as "Thavil Kattai" in Tamil or "Dolu Tantram" in Telugu. This replica of the Thavil consists of a treble side and a bass side. On the bass side, a sponge is glued to the wood, allowing the student to strike it with a stick. The treble side is covered with plain wood and animal skin, simulating the actual drumhead. Initially, students practice without wearing the rings or caps on their fingers, focusing on basic lessons.
Since practice involves striking bare fingers on a hard wooden surface, it gradually toughens the fingers, but can also cause blisters on the phalanx of each finger and swelling of the upper part of the palm. Despite the discomfort, this training strengthens the hands, preparing students for playing on the actual Thavil.

Rings, Caps, and Stick

I. When playing the real Thavil, the performer wears rings and caps on their fingers to strike the treble drumhead. However, prolonged use of these rings and caps can cause abrasion and discomfort, leading to pain. To prevent this, it is advisable to wrap a small piece of cloth around the fingertips before placing the caps, providing both protection and a secure fit for the caps on the fingers.

II. While playing on the bass head of the Thavil, the player uses a stick to strike the drumhead. However, holding the stick continuously for 3 h can cause swelling in the palm, leading to discomfort and fatigue.

Ergonomics of the Instrument

I. The Thavil is a double-sided drum consisting of a wooden frame and animal skin drumheads, with an approximate weight of 13–15 kg. In modern designs, the use of bolts and nuts to secure the drumheads to the shell increases the weight by an additional 2–3 kg. As a result, placing a 15 kg instrument on the lap and practicing for several hours can cause muscle cramps and leg pain. The pressure exerted on the ankle may also lead to swelling, making prolonged practice physically demanding.

II. The Thavil is known as "Mangal Vadyam," meaning an instrument suitable for processions. One of the most common injuries associated with playing the Thavil is back and neck pain, caused by carrying the heavy instrument while walking and playing simultaneously. During long temple processions, performers must carry the Thavil and play continuously for 2–3 h, placing significant strain on the shoulders, spine, and neck. Over time, this prolonged stress can lead to postural issues, including a hunched back, making it a physically demanding practice.

C. In the Case of a Ghatam player:

Materials of the Instrument

I. There are three main types of Ghatams: the "Madras Ghatam" from Chennai, the "Devanahalli Ghatam" from Bangalore, and the most renowned "Manamadurai Ghatam" from Manamadurai. The Manamadurai Ghatam is the most widely used due to its superior sound quality compared to the others.
   However, a key disadvantage of the Manamadurai Ghatams is that it is made from a specific type of clay found in that region, resulting in a thicker instrument. The increased thickness makes it more challenging to play and practice. Prolonged practice sessions on these Ghatams can cause the hands to harden and develop blisters, which may eventually tear and lead to abrasions on the fingertips.
II. While playing bass notes on the Ghatam, the player strikes the lower part of the palm (on the wrist crease) against the thick, solid surface of the instrument. This repeated impact can lead to swelling and hardening on the wrist crease over time.

10.2 Ergonomics of the Instrument

I. The Ghatam has a solid structure and typically weighs between 5 and 8 kg, with the Manamadurai Ghatam weighing around 7–8 kg. Keeping an 8 kg Ghatam on the lap for extended periods, whether during practice or concerts lasting 2–3 h, can cause discomfort, leading to muscle pain and cramps in the thighs and legs.

D. In the Case of a Kanjira Player: *Material of the Instrument*
   I. The frame of the Kanjira is made of wood, hence holding a wooden frame for a long period can cause pain in muscles, fatigue, and strain in the palm of the non-dominant hand.
   II. The side of the proximal phalanx of the thumb is made of soft skin; hence, continuous friction against the wooden frame can lead to skin abrasions and discomfort.
   III. The skin of the drumhead of the Kanjira is made up of the Bengal monitor lizard skin, which is moderately hard; hence, repetitive impact on the index finger and the palm can lead to blisters and swelling over time.

Ergonomics of the Instrument

I. The width of the Kanjira frame is approximately 2–3 inches; hence, bending the thumb inward and securing the 3-inch frame with the fingers and the palm can lead to swelling on the palm and pain near the base of the thumb over time.
   It is known that if we hold something too big for our hand for a long period, we can experience discomfort, strain in the hand and arm muscles, potential loss of grip, and even drop the object. Hence, artists with smaller hands often experience greater difficulty holding the 3-inch frame, as it exceeds their natural grip capacity, leading to fatigue and discomfort during prolonged play.

E. In the Case of a Morsing Player: *Material of the Instrument*
   I. The entire instrument is made of metal with sharp edges. The frame/bridge is made of iron, while the middle rod and reed are made of steel. As a result, placing the instrument in the mouth may cause minor injuries to the gums.
   II. Additionally, holding the metal frame between the teeth can lead to corrosion, increasing the risk of tooth sensitivity and decay.
   III. According to some artists, since the middle rod is made of steel, placing the

tongue on it while it vibrates may cause tongue lacerations.

IV. When plucking the metal reed that extends outside the mouth, it may strike the side of the lip, leading to swelling, tears, and bleeding.

V. Furthermore, since the metal reed is as sharp as a blade, continuous plucking can cause abrasions on the tip of the index or middle finger.

F. In the Case of a Tabla Player: *Drumhead Materials*:

I. The drumheads of the Tabla are normally made of goat skin, stretched tightly over the shell using leather straps and wooden pegs to produce its soft, harmonic tone. However, continuous finger strikes on the taut treble drumhead can cause blisters to develop on the phalanges.

II. The drumhead skins are tightly secured with leather straps, braided along the edges, known as *Gajra*. While playing, the upper part of the palm repeatedly strikes the *Gajra* causing blisters. Over time, these blisters harden and develop into permanent calluses on the palm.

III. Tabla artists are prone to developing bruises on the wrist crease due to the continuous back-and-forth sliding motion required to create modulation bass sound effects. The repeated pressure and friction on the wrist can lead to bruising the persistent pain over time.

11 Repetitive Strain due to Prolonged Practice Sessions

A. In the Matter of a Mridangam Player:

Arm Movement

I. Injuries such as tendons and muscle strains in the shoulder and elbow may occur due to prolonged practice sessions. While analyzing the hand movement, we can notice that abduction and adduction movements take place, resulting in pain in the shoulders, elbows, and muscles in this area.

We must note that the forearm is perpendicular to the upper arm, for the hand playing the treble hand; hence, this can result in muscle strains in the upper arm and the forearm.

Sitting Posture

I. Mridangam is usually practiced while sitting down cross-legged. Pain such as lower back pain can occur due to long sitting down and practicing for hours.

B. In the Matter of a Thavil Player: *Wrist Movement*

I. As explained earlier, a stick is used to strike the bass head of the Thavil. While playing, the non-dominant wrist undergoes radial and ulnar deviation movements, while the dominant wrist performs frequent flexion and extension movements to help the caps on the fingers strike the drumhead. Repeating these movements for extended practice sessions can strain the wrist tendons, leading to pain and discomfort.

Arm Movement

I. While standing and playing the Thavil, greater muscle strength is required. The non-dominant upper arm undergoes abduction and adduction movements, while the dominant forearm performs similar motions. These repetitive movements can lead to joint pain in the elbow and shoulder over time.

II. Moreover, continuous hand movements during prolonged performances cause muscle fatigue, resulting in pain in the forearm and upper arm, making standing play physically demanding.

Sitting Posture

I. Sitting cross-legged while supporting the heavy Thavil on the leg can lead to muscle pain and cramps, making prolonged practice physically challenging.

Standing Posture

I. Standing for long hours while holding the heavy Thavil can cause pain in the lower back and hips. To reduce strain, many players now use a Thavil stand, which supports the instrument during extended standing performances, allowing for greater comfort and endurance.

C. In the Matter of a Ghatam Player: *Arm Movement*
   I. While playing the Ghatam, the upper arm remains straight, while the forearm is raised in a "guard position." Continuous up-and-down movements of the forearm are required to strike the instrument. These repetitive motions can lead to tendon inflammation in the elbows, especially when kept tucked, and may also cause stiffness in the shoulders.
   Additionally, these arm movements can result in muscle pain in both the upper arm and forearm of both hands.
   II. Moreover, as explained earlier, various techniques are used to produce the bass sound effect, such as striking the lower palm of the left hand against the instrument or hitting the mouth of the Ghatam with the entire palm. These repetitive movements can lead to bruises and abrasions under the wrist, as well as swelling from prolonged practice sessions.
   Additionally, the wrist may experience tendon pain due to these continuous motions.

Sitting Posture

I. To create effects such as the *Gumki*, the player must tilt their abdomen forward and backward, pressing it against the opening of the Ghatam. Repeating this motion for extended practice sessions can strain the spine and cause back pain.
II. Holding the heavy Ghatam on the lap for long hours can restrict blood circulation, potentially leading to cramps in the legs.

D. In the Matter of a Kanjira Player: *Arm Movement*
   I. While playing the Kanjira, the dominant hand undergoes continuous abduction and adduction movements in the forearm. Hence, prolonged practice can lead to tendon pain in the wrist and elbow, as well as a muscle strain in the forearm and deltoid muscles near the shoulder.
   II. On the other hand, keeping the non-dominant hand forearm perpendicular and holding the instrument for an extended period can cause muscle strain on the forearm and the upper arm muscles.

Sitting Posture

I. The Kanjira player usually sits down cross-legged on the ground and practices for hours, and this leads to lower back pain, hip stiffness, and pain in the thigh muscle, which can lead to cramps.
II. Poor posture or imbalance while sitting can create uneven strain on the spine, shoulders, and arms, leading to discomfort and long-term posture-related issues.

E. In the Matter of a Morsing Player: *Wrist Movement*
   I. Due to repetitive radial and ulnar deviation movements of the wrist, the player may experience tendon pain in the dominant hand from plucking the metal reed during long practice hours.

Holding the Instrument

I. Holding the instrument with the non-dominant hand for a long time can cause joint pain in the wrist and elbow. This is because the wrist remains in a fixed straight position while the elbow stays tucked to keep the forearm raised near the mouth.
II. Maintaining the arm in a "guard position" for an extended period can cause muscle pain in the upper arm and forearm.

Sitting Posture

I. Prolonged sitting and practice in a cross-legged position can cause cramps and discomfort in the Morsing player's legs.

F. In the Matter of a Tabla Player: *Wrist Movement*
   I. Tabla players rely heavily on wrist movements to ensure precise finger strikes on the upward-facing drumheads. This constant motion can lead to tendon strain and joint pain in the wrist over time.
   II. Further, the repetitive movements can cause discomfort or pain in the extensor carpi radialis brevis muscle of the forearm.

Sitting Posture

I. Tabla players typically practice while seated in a cross-legged position for extended periods. Prolonged sitting can lead to lower back pain and spinal stiffness, resulting in discomfort and potential postural issues over time.

II. Like other musicians who practice in a seated position, Tabla players often experience cramps from prolonged cross-legged sitting during extended practice sessions.

12 Poor Posture or Improper Technique

A. Regarding a Mridangam Player: *Arm Positioning*

I. The upper arm should be positioned at an angle of approximately 30° relative to the ribs. Poor posture can lead to arm pain and injury, especially when students extend the upper arm too far outward or raise the elbow too high. This incorrect positioning can strain the shoulders and elbows, resulting in discomfort or pain over time.

II. Arm pain, including muscle strains and tendon discomfort around the elbow, often arises from improper arm movements while playing the Mridangam. Adopting specific wrist movements during practice is generally more effective and efficient for handling the instrument. In contrast, relying heavily on elbow or shoulder movements can increase strain on the muscles and joints, potentially leading to pain or injury over time.

Sitting Posture

I. While sitting cross-legged and practicing, some students and performers tend to lean their torso forward toward the Mridangam. This posture causes the spine to bend slightly, which, over time, can lead to back pain due to the constant strain on the spinal cord. Prolonged practice in a bent position may even result in a hunched back if the habit persists without correction.

II. Additionally, excessive bending of the spine can cause the neck to bend as well, leading to discomfort such as axial neck pain.

B. Regarding a Thavil Player: *Arm Positioning*

I. In the seated posture, the player's forearm should remain perpendicular to the upper arm, with the elbow positioned neither too far nor too close to the body. Incorrect positioning can lead to joint pain in the elbow and shoulder, as well as muscle strain in the shoulder and upper arm.

Standing Posture

I. While standing and playing, the player should avoid bending the torso toward the instrument while carrying it. Poor posture can lead to back and neck pain and is one of the reasons why some Thavil artists develop a hunchback over time.

C. Regarding a Ghatam: *Arm Positioning*

I. The elbow is usually kept close to the body of the performer. However, if the player extends the elbow to help the forearm strike the instrument, it can strain the tendons, leading to pain in the elbows and shoulders.

Sitting Posture

I. While pressing the mouth of the Ghatam with the stomach, the player pushes their torso forward, which can lead to back and neck pain. To reduce excessive forward and backward bending, modern techniques have been introduced. One such technique involves widening the legs and positioning the Ghatam lower between the thighs. By moving the thighs in a butterfly motion, the instrument itself moves forward and backward, minimizing the need for the player to shift their body.

D. Regarding a Morsing Player: *Neck and Back Position*

I. While practicing, some artists have a habit of pushing their neck forward, which can lead to axial neck pain.

II. Moreover, sitting in the lotus posture with a bent back can cause spinal discomfort, leading to back pain.

Elbow Position

I. If the elbow of the dominant hand is positioned too far from the body, it can cause muscle pain in the arm. To prevent this, the elbow should remain close to the body in a natural position.

Breathing Technique

I. While playing the Morsing, the player needs to inhale and exhale continuously to sustain the vibration of the sound. However, rapid breathing can cause hyperventilation syndrome, leading to shortness of breath, chest pain, dizziness, and other discomforts.

E. Regarding a Tabla Player: *Arm Positioning*

   I. Both hands are normally positioned on the Tabla, with the forearm extended at approximately 160° to the upper arms and the elbow facing downward. However, some players develop a habit of lifting their elbows outward, which results in muscle strain in the shoulders and upper arms, as well as joint pain in the elbows due to improper posture.

Sitting Posture

I. While sitting cross-legged, some players tend to slouch or bend their backs, which can result in lower back pain and stiffness in the spinal cord over time.

II. Moreover, some players experience axial neck pain due to improper forward bending of the neck while practicing.

13 Posture and Technique-Related Issues

- Improper *arm positioning*, *elbow elevation*, and *spine bending* result in pain and chronic conditions (Workman 2003).
- Seated posture without back support contributes to spinal and neck pain (Haas 2003).
- Breathing control in Morsing is critical to avoid dizziness (Workman 2013).

14 Impact of One-Handed Playing (Especially for a Kanjira Player)

I. Unlike most percussion instruments that utilize both hands, the Kanjira relies entirely on one hand for playing, placing excessive strain on the dominant arm. Over time, this can lead to muscle stiffness and fatigue. Additionally, since the non-dominant hand primarily holds the instrument, it does not develop the same level of strength and flexibility, resulting in muscle imbalance between the two arms.

15 Mental Fatigue

A. For a Kanjira Player:

   I. Another challenge is mental fatigue. Since a Kanjira player must replicate rhythms that other percussionists play with two hands using only one, it demands intense focus, rapid execution, and greater precision. The fast-paced strokes required can generate friction burns, leading to blisters and abrasions, while the constant mental effort can cause cognitive exhaustion over time.

B. For a Morsing Player:

   I. Nevertheless, the Morsing player experiences mental fatigue, as the art requires intense focus. The artist must manage breathing while plucking and vocalizing, ensuring they do not injure any part of the mouth, such as the tongue. Some artists feel significant fatigue in the head after a concert or prolonged practice session.

16 Conclusion

Indian percussion instruments—while diverse in design and technique—pose a range of physiological and ergonomic challenges. Musicians are susceptible to skin trauma, muscle overuse, tendon inflammation, joint strain, postural injuries, and even mental fatigue due to prolonged, high-intensity practice sessions. Prevention includes ergonomic redesigns, postural correction, muscle strengthening, and guided practice routines. Educators and health professionals must remain vigilant to preserve both performance quality and physical wellbeing of percussionists.

References

Haas K (2003) Coping with a playing related injury. Percussive Notes, December, p 50

Harnsberger A (2008) Stretching for pain-free performance. Percussive Notes, February, pp 54–56

May D (1994) Injury prevention in percussion. Percussive Notes, April, pp 73–75

McKinney J (2010) The secret to injury prevention. Percussive Notes, May, pp 12–13

Molina O (2018) How to stay in the game: percussion injury prevention and treatment. National conference on Percussion Pedagogy, University of Arkansas, May.

Paris N (1995) Performing arts medicine. Percussive Notes, October, p 64

Workman D (1999) Injury prevention: the teacher's responsibility. Percussive Notes, June, pp 57–60

Workman D (2003) Carpal tunnel syndrome: ignoring the symptoms that can end your career. Percussive Notes, June, pp 8–13

Workman D (2013) The percussionist's guide to injury treatment and prevention: the answer guide to drummers in pain. Taylor and Francis, Florence

Ergonomics of a Musician

Veenadhari Bhamidipaty, Urvashi Mohinani,
and Kanaka Durga Prasad Bhamidipaty

Contents

V. Bhamidipaty
Department of CSE, GITAM, Visakhapatnam, India

U. Mohinani
Department of Fine & Performing Arts, GITAM, Visakhapatnam, India

K. D. P. Bhamidipaty (✉)
Department of Radiodiagnosis, NRIIMS, Visakhapatnam, India

Med Radiol Diagn Imaging (2025)

https://doi.org/10.1007/174_2025_626,
Published Online: 25 September 2025

Abstract

This document explores the critical role of ergonomics in preventing musculoskeletal injuries among musicians, emphasizing the physical demands of playing various instruments and the importance of proper technique, posture, and practice habits. It examines the prevalence and risk factors of playing-related musculoskeletal disorders (PRMDs), such as carpal tunnel syndrome, tendinitis, and focal dystonia, which affect 26%–93% of instrumental musicians. Instrument-specific ergonomic challenges for keyboardists, string players, wind instrumentalists, percussionists, and vocalists are analyzed, alongside preventive strategies including postural adjustments, warm-up routines, and workload management. The integration of ergonomic principles into music education is highlighted as essential for fostering sustainable careers. By synthesizing research from performing arts medicine, this work underscores the need for musicians and educators to prioritize ergonomic awareness to enhance performance longevity and artistic expression while minimizing injury risks.

1 Introduction

Ergonomics is the discipline that aligns working circumstances and task requirements with the worker's capabilities. This information aims to give musicians and their supervisors a fundamental comprehension of ergonomics and instrumental injuries and highlight supervisors' crucial role in preventing these injuries. It is important to note that instrumental injuries frequently encompass the same ailments associated with excessive computer use. This shared risk underscores the need for all of us, musicians and computer users alike, to be mindful of our ergonomic practices.

These injuries, including carpal tunnel syndrome, tendinitis, bursitis, tenosynovitis/De Quervain's syndrome, tendinosis, thoracic outlet syndrome, myofascial pain syndrome, cubital tunnel syndrome, and trigger finger/thumb, are notably prevalent among keyboardists, fretboardists, flutists, and string instrumentalists. It is crucial that we all, as musicians and supervisors, are aware of these risks. Improper posture, non-ergonomic methods, excessive exertion, overuse, stress, and inadequate rest lead to chronic injuries that may result in significant discomfort, potential disability, and job termination.

Over the past 25 years, it has been clear that musicians are at risk for harm. Concerns regarding the possibility of injury have been increasingly prevalent in the music industry. Studies in performing arts medicine indicate that roughly 25% of music students suffer from playing-related injuries, a statistic that underscores the severity of the issue (Zaza 1998). Years of a professional musician's life are dedicated to practicing, frequently calling for exact and repeated motions. This environment significantly contributes to the prevalence of overuse injuries (PRMD/PRP) among instrumental players (Ackermann and Adams 2004a). The practice duration of a musician presents particular challenges in elucidation. However, through rigorous research, we have understood that extended practice durations without breaks and individuals who practice for several hours daily are linked to PRMD/PRP (Baadjou et al. 2016). No study delineated the specific number of practice hours per day that constituted a risk threshold; nonetheless, multiple studies indicated that consistent practice sessions above 1.5–2 h were correlated with PRMD/PRP (Baadjou et al. 2016). Numerous reviewed publications suggest that age correlates with an elevated risk of PRMD/PRP; nevertheless, this observation does not apply exclusively to older artists. Reviewed articles indicate a correlation between PRMD/PRP and both young/adolescent musicians and older musicians, in contrast to middle-aged musicians (Ranelli et al. 2014).

The definition of bad ergonomics when playing varies according to the instrument. Recognizing the importance of objective assessment, various tools (such as the Rapid Upper Limb Assessment Tool) have been proposed to provide data on artists' methods contributing to PRMD/PRP (Berque et al. 2016). These tools play a crucial role in identifying and preventing injuries, underscoring their significance in the field of musician health.

Musicians' musculoskeletal injuries are intricately linked to their practice habits. This is where the pivotal role of music educators comes into play. They not only can, but must, assume a crucial role in injury prevention, empowering them with a sense of responsibility and the ability to make a significant impact.

In 2003, the National Association of Schools of Music (NASM), the accrediting organization for degree-granting music institutions in the United States, made a significant statement in its handbook. It emphasized that institutions should facilitate students' acquisition of knowledge from qualified professionals and authoritative medical sources concerning the maintenance of professional health and the prevention of performance-related injuries (Guptill and Zaza 2010). The statement also highlighted the grave consequences of chronic injuries, such as significant pain, potential injury or disability, and a breakdown of careers, underscoring the gravity of the situation. The absence of a warm-up before practice, rehearsal, or performance was linked to the onset of PRMD/PRP. Baadjou et al. (2016) discovered that warm-up safeguards against the first PRMD; however, no study specified what constitutes sufficient warm-up duration. Focal dystonia is an idiopathic hyperkinetic movement disease that may impact any skeletal muscle. Dystonia in musicians is task-specific and is dreaded by musicians as it often signifies the conclusion of their musical career (Brandfonbrener 2009a). Musicians may encounter musculoskeletal issues due to their profession significantly differ according to the instrument they play.

Work-related musculoskeletal disorders (WMSDs) are not just injuries or diseases affecting muscles, nerves, tendons, joints, cartilage, and spinal discs. They are significant health issues that can severely impact the lives of musicians, both professionally and personally. These disorders, characterized by their work-related causation or exacerbation, can lead to limitations in both occupational and non-occupational activities. The literature indicates that the lifetime prevalence of WMSDs among professional musicians is high, ranging from 62% to 93% (Zaza and Farewell 1997). Musculoskeletal diseases or injuries associated with playing activities can differ according to the type of instrument utilized. For instance, Paarup et al. (2011) have discovered that musicians performing in orchestras often experience discomfort in their necks, shoulders, and backs, affecting their daily lives and performance. Static muscle activity in a specific instrumental position frequently causes excessive elongation of the tendons and joints, leading to musculoskeletal pain. Prolonged instrument playing poses the risk of chronic pain syndrome development. Chronic pain is typically associated with neuromuscular alterations. These factors may jeopardize musicians' professional careers (Ackermann et al. 2012).

Performance-related WMSDs are not solely a result of static muscle activity. They stem from a complex interaction between the instrument and the musician. Extrinsic aspects, such as the musician's technique and the performance setting, play a significant role in their development (Chan and Ackermann 2014). As the scientific study of job design, ergonomics is not just about understanding the human body's capabilities and limitations. Its objective is to proactively mitigate the dangers employees encounter throughout their jobs by properly designing work equipment, thereby reducing the risk of musculoskeletal issues and enhancing work performance.

2 The Relationship Between Musicianship and Ergonomics

Musicianship is a multifaceted discipline that demands a seamless integration of technical proficiency, expressive artistry, and physical endurance. The repetitive and physically intensive nature of instrumental performance places significant demands on the musculoskeletal system, requiring sustained precision, agility, and coordination. Without a comprehensive understanding of ergonomics, musicians risk developing chronic musculoskeletal strain, fatigue-related injuries, and biomechanical inefficiencies, which can compromise performance quality and career longevity (Horvath 2010).

By embracing ergonomic principles, musicians can take control of their postural alignment, physical stress, and neuromuscular coordination. This control leads to greater technical control, expressive range, and endurance. Aligning instrumental technique with biomechanical efficiency empowers musicians to cultivate sustainable playing habits, mitigate injury risks, and foster refined precision, enhanced tonal control, and fluid expressivity. An ergonomically sound approach is the foundation for artistic mastery and professional longevity, ensuring musicians can engage with their craft at the highest level while preserving their physical well-being and performance resilience.

2.1 Ergonomics and Technical Proficiency in Musicianship

Ergonomics directly impacts a musician's ability to develop, refine, and sustain technical proficiency, endurance, and artistic control. Inefficient body mechanics—such as poor posture, improper hand positioning, excessive muscular tension, and repetitive overuse—can hinder fluid movement, reduce agility, limit dynamic range, and increase the risk of strain-related injuries (Horvath 2010). By integrating ergonomically sound techniques, musicians can optimize their efficiency, comfort, and performance longevity, ensuring sustainable artistic growth.

2.1.1 Posture (Physical Demands) and Playing Efficiency

Postural alignment is not just a good habit; it is foundational to playing efficiency, breath control, endurance, and coordination. An ergonomically balanced sitting or standing posture ensures that musicians engage the appropriate muscle groups while minimizing unnecessary tension and fatigue (Ackermann and Adams 2004b). Maintaining a neutral spinal position and proper weight distribution promotes stability and biomechanical efficiency, allowing unrestricted movement and enhanced control.

However, poor postural habits—such as slouching, excessive arching, or asymmetrical weight distribution—can cause muscular compensation, leading to chronic back pain, shoulder stiffness, joint misalignment, and reduced endurance (Brandfonbrener 2009b). For instrumentalists, specific postural considerations include the following:

- *String instruments (e.g., violin, guitar)*: Requires intricate finger work and sustained arm positioning, posing risks of shoulder and wrist strain without proper support.
- *Wind Instruments (e.g., flute, clarinet)*: Demands controlled breathing, finger dexterity, and posture alignment, which can lead to back and neck discomfort if not managed ergonomically.
- *Percussion Instruments (e.g., drum, tabla)*: Involves repetitive, high-impact motions that can strain wrists, elbows, and shoulders.
- *Keyboard Instruments (e.g., piano, organ)*: Necessitates balanced hand positioning and wrist alignment to prevent overuse injuries.
- *Vocal ergonomics*: Challenges include managing breath control, maintaining an upright posture, and avoiding vocal strain during prolonged singing.

Preventive Strategies

- Maintain neutral spinal alignment to promote efficient weight distribution.
- For instance, a wind instrumentalist might benefit from a chair with a backrest that supports a straight spine, while a percussionist could use a drum throne with adjustable height and a padded seat to distribute weight evenly.
- Regularly assess and adjust posture to prevent muscle fatigue and tension buildup.

2.1.2 Hand and Finger Dexterity

Dexterity in hand and finger movements is critical for precision, agility, and speed in musicianship. Ergonomic awareness in hand positioning, wrist alignment, and muscle relaxation is essential to prevent injuries caused by excessive force, rigid grip, or awkward angles. Overuse syndromes such as tendinitis, carpal tunnel syndrome, and tenosynovitis are common among musicians who neglect proper biomechanical techniques (Zaza 1998).

- *Keyboard Players*: Wrists should remain neutral, preventing excessive flexion or extension that could compress the median nerve.
- *String Players*: The left-hand fingers should curve naturally, ensuring smooth fingerboard navigation, while the right-hand bowing motion should be fluid and relaxed (Horvath 2010).
- *Percussionists*: Wrist flexibility and rebound control should be coordinated, minimizing shock absorption strain and avoiding excessive wrist flexion (Chan and Ackermann 2014).

Preventive Strategies
- Keep wrists relaxed and maintain a natural curvature in the fingers.
- For example, a pianist could do finger stretches by placing their hand flat on a table and gently pressing each finger down, one at a time. This helps to improve finger strength and flexibility.
- Avoid forceful gripping and excessive muscular tension during playing.

2.2 Impact of Ergonomics on Musical Expression

2.2.1 Breath Control and Body Mechanics

For wind and brass players, breath control is fundamental in producing a resonant tone, executing dynamic contrast, and sustaining phrases. Ergonomic awareness ensures that ribcage expansion, diaphragm engagement, and airflow regulation remain unrestricted, preventing unnecessary tension that could compromise tone quality and endurance (Ackermann and Adams 2004b).

However, poor postural alignment and excess muscular engagement in the neck, shoulders, and jaw can impede lung function, leading to inconsistent airflow, diminished breath support, and reduced tonal flexibility.

Common Postural Challenges Affecting Breath Control
- *Collapsed Chest & Slouching*: Limits lung expansion, reducing airflow capacity and dynamic range.
- *Tension in Neck & Shoulders*: Restricts laryngeal movement, affecting tone modulation and flexibility.
- *Rigid Jaw & Tongue Positioning*: Disrupts articulation and resonance, leading to poor tonal clarity.

Preventive Strategies
- Maintain an open chest posture to facilitate free diaphragmatic movement and lung expansion.
- Engage in deep breathing exercises to enhance breath endurance and airflow consistency.
- Avoid excessive neck and jaw tension, ensuring relaxed, efficient breathing mechanics.

2.2.2 Freedom of Movement and Expressivity

Musical expression is not just about technical precision but also about the fluidity of movement that allows for natural phrasing, articulation, and dynamic control. Excessive physical rigidity or compensatory muscular tension can significantly inhibit expressiveness, making performances feel mechanical and restricted (Horvath 2010).

Each instrumentalist requires unrestricted, well-coordinated movements to shape their sound effectively:

- *String Players*: A relaxed bowing arm enhances legato phrasing, dynamic shading, and tonal variation.
- *Keyboardists*: Proper wrist flexibility and forearm rotation allow smooth phrasing, articulation, and expressiveness.
- *Percussionists*: Efficient wrist rebound control minimizes unnecessary muscular effort, ensuring fluidity in rhythmic execution.

Preventive Strategies

- Use balanced muscle engagement rather than excessive force to facilitate unrestricted movement.
- Incorporate body awareness techniques (e.g., Alexander Technique, Feldenkrais Method) to refine movement efficiency and reduce tension.
- Ensure adequate warm-ups before playing to promote relaxed, controlled motion.

2.3 Injury Prevention and Longevity in Musicianship

The sustainability of a musician's career depends heavily on preventing musculoskeletal disorders, which can arise from repetitive overuse, poor posture, and improper playing techniques. Many injuries associated with instrumental performance develop gradually, making early intervention and ergonomic awareness essential.

2.3.1 Repetitive Strain Injuries (RSIs)

RSIs occur when repetitive motions—such as finger movements, wrist flexion, or prolonged static postures—lead to muscle fatigue, tendon inflammation, and nerve compression (Guptill and Zaza 2010). If left unaddressed, these conditions can become chronic and career-threatening.

Common RSIs in Musicians

- *Carpal Tunnel Syndrome*: Caused by extended wrist flexion, which results in finger weakness, tingling, and numbness (Zaza and Farewell 1997).
- *Tendinitis & Tenosynovitis*: The overuse of the flexor and extensor tendons leads to inflammation and stiffness (Chan and Ackermann 2014).
- *Thoracic Outlet Syndrome*: Overly raised arms and tense shoulders can compress blood vessels and nerves, resulting in discomfort, tingling, and problems with circulation (Horvath 2010).

Preventive Strategies

- Implement frequent micro-breaks to prevent cumulative fatigue and overuse injuries.
- Perform targeted stretching and strengthening exercises to maintain muscular flexibility and endurance.
- Maintain neutral wrist and arm positioning to minimize tendon strain and nerve compression.

By integrating ergonomic principles into daily practice, musicians can reduce injury risks, improve technical efficiency, and enhance artistic freedom, ensuring a long, sustainable career in performance.

2.3.2 Postural Imbalances and Fatigue

Musicians often maintain static postures for extended periods, which, if not properly managed, can result in muscular imbalances, joint compression, and chronic pain. Sustained poor posture not only affects technical performance and endurance but can also have a significant impact on a musician's career, potentially leading to long-term musculoskeletal disorders (Zaza and Farewell 1997).

When the body is consistently positioned out of alignment, specific muscle groups overcompensate, while others become weakened or restricted. This can lead to postural asymmetry, excessive joint strain, and nerve compression, affecting playing efficiency and overall well-being.

2.3.2.1 Common Postural Challenges Across Different Instrumentalists

Keyboardists: Forward Head Posture and Upper Back Stiffness

Keyboard players often spend hours practicing in a seated position, frequently looking down at sheet music or keys. This can result in forward head posture (FHP)—a condition where the head is positioned too far forward relative to the shoulders, increasing strain on the cervical spine and upper back muscles.

Effects of Forward Head Posture in Keyboardists

- Increased neck and upper back tension due to prolonged isometric muscle contraction.
- Restricted shoulder mobility, affecting fluid arm movement and playing efficiency.
- Compression of cervical vertebrae leads to headaches, stiffness, and nerve impingement.

Preventive Strategies for Keyboardists

- Maintain a neutral head position by aligning the ears with the shoulders.
- Adjust the music stand height to eye level to prevent excessive neck flexion.
- Perform neck retraction and upper back strengthening exercises to counteract FHP.

String Players: Uneven Shoulder Elevation and Muscular Imbalance

String musicians, especially violinists and violists, often experience muscular asymmetry due to uneven shoulder positioning while holding their instruments. The left shoulder remains elevated to support the instrument, while the right arm engages in repetitive bowing motions, causing muscle overuse and imbalance.

Effects of Uneven Shoulder Elevation in String Players

- Overdeveloped trapezius and levator scapulae muscles on one side, leading to postural misalignment.
- Increased neck and upper back strain, contributing to stiffness and discomfort.
- Potential nerve compression in the shoulder girdle, leading to numbness or tingling in the arms.

Preventive Strategies for String Players

- Regularly alternate shoulder stretches to maintain muscular balance.
- Use ergonomic shoulder rests and chin rests to distribute instrument weight evenly.
- Engage in postural awareness exercises like the Alexander Technique to minimize unnecessary tension.

Percussionists: Cross-Legged Seating, Knee Stiffness, and Hip Misalignment

Percussionists, especially those playing Indian classical instruments like tabla or mridangam, often sit cross-legged for extended durations. This posture can lead to hip flexor tightness, knee compression, and lower back discomfort due to an uneven weight distribution and prolonged static positioning.

Effects of Cross-Legged Sitting in Percussionists

- Limited hip mobility, resulting in stiffness and discomfort over time.
- Increased knee compression, potentially leading to joint pain or restricted circulation.
- Asymmetrical spinal loading, causing misalignment and lower back discomfort.

Preventive Strategies for Percussionists

- Use a small cushion or yoga block under the hips to maintain spinal neutrality.
- Regularly shift leg positions or extend the legs intermittently to relieve stiffness.
- Engage in hip mobility exercises and lower body stretches to prevent joint compression.

2.3.2.2 General Postural Correction and Injury Prevention Strategies

Musicians should incorporate postural realignment exercises and ergonomic adjustments into their daily practice routines to mitigate the risks associated with sustained poor posture.

Comprehensive Preventive Strategies

- Maintaining an upright, balanced posture with proper spinal support ensures even weight distribution.
- Adjust instrument height and positioning according to individual comfort and biomechanical efficiency.
- Engage in postural realignment exercises (e.g., core strengthening, flexibility drills, and myofascial release techniques) to counteract imbalances and tension buildup.

By integrating ergonomics and body awareness into practice routines, musicians can enhance endurance, reduce injury risks, and improve performance longevity. These strategies ensure both technical precision and physical well-being, giving musicians a positive outlook on their future in the industry.

3 Physical Injuries Among Musicians

When it comes to injuries, the two most prevalent types are back problems and cumulative trauma disorders (also known as CTD). Workplace awareness and responsibility are not just important; they are crucial to preventing these. Back disorders are frequently caused by muscles, ligaments, tendons, and disks that have been pulled or stretched. It is crucial to be aware of the symptoms and seek early detection. Lifting or carrying loads that are overly heavy, twisting, or remaining in an awkward position for extended periods are all potential contributing factors that can lead to these injuries. Backaches and an inability to raise or move around are two of the symptoms that may be experienced.

Cumulative trauma illnesses can affect various parts of the body, including the upper and lower arms, elbows, wrists, hands and fingers, shoulders and neck, lower limbs, and back. They are often linked to activities that involve repeated motion over a prolonged period in conjunction with uncomfortable posture or force. A tingling or numbing sensation may be experienced in the palms, fingers, or other parts of the body as one of the symptoms being experienced.

Other symptoms include discomfort or pain and difficulties moving the fingers, shoulders, elbows, wrists, or backs with the affected hand.

These injuries can have a significant impact on a musician's career, making it crucial to be aware of and take precautions against upper extremity injuries, including those affecting the hand, arm, and shoulder. This includes overuse injuries, strains and sprains, inflammatory disorders (e.g., tendonitis, tenosynovitis), nerve compression syndromes (e.g., carpal tunnel syndrome), and additional neurological illnesses, such as focal dystonia. Instrumentalists also exhibit symptoms in the back and neck. However, these have been less thoroughly documented in the literature on performing arts medicine. Temporomandibular joint disorder, impacting the articulations between the jaw and skull, may cause worry for specific individuals, while others might encounter dermatological conditions (e.g., violinists' neck). Musicians may also experience significant performance anxiety and various mental health issues.

The reported prevalence rates of playing-related injuries among instrumental musicians are alarmingly high, ranging from 26% to 93% (Zaza 1998). The true prevalence of these issues within the musician community is challenging to ascertain due to the lack of fully established processes for definitive diagnoses. Moreover, significant disparities exist in the incidence of specific injury types among various common instrument categories (piano, upper strings, guitar, flute, other woodwinds, and percussion).

4 Determinants of Injury Risk

Playing is associated with a significant risk factor. Using repetitive motions over a lengthy period during practice is one of the factors that can lead to injuries. In particular, musicians are more likely to get injuries when they experience a sudden rise in their time practicing. Whether you are preparing for a significant audition or performance or starting your studies in professional music, sudden increases in practice time can be a red flag for potential injuries. Stress and worry are risk factors in obtaining injuries, making managing these factors and your practice schedule crucial. Furthermore, it has been demonstrated that stress affects performance (Sapir et al. 1994). The awkward body positions required by the instrument's form and weight, the repertoire's technical difficulties, and playing instruments foreign to the player are all potential factors that might ultimately lead to injury. The total number of years spent playing is also a risk factor for ailments associated with playing.

Factors contributing to playing-related injuries include gender (women appear to be at greater risk than males) and the instrument played. String players and pianists have elevated injury rates, with age and body mass index (BMI) indicating that older musicians and those with a higher BMI face an augmented risk of injury (Furuya et al. 2014). Moreover, hypermobility (double-jointedness) may constitute a risk factor; however, it is crucial to acknowledge that hypermobility is more prevalent among musicians than in the general population. The correlation between hypermobility and injuries remains ambiguous. However, many factors contributing to playing-related injuries are associated with playing behaviors, which are subject to modification. This suggests that there is potential for change and improvement. Students can be instructed in beneficial playing habits that may aid in preventing future injuries. Consequently, it is essential for educators not only to instruct pupils on what to practice but also to demonstrate the practice methods (Guptill and Zaza 2010).

The cumulative years of instrument playing also significantly determine playing-related musculoskeletal disorders (PRMDs). Research indicates that musicians with extensive playing experience are at greater risk of chronic strain injuries due to prolonged exposure to repetitive movements (Ranelli et al. 2014). Long-term playing leads to repetitive stress on the musculoskeletal system, particularly in regions such as the wrists, shoulders, and spine. The continued use of improper playing techniques can further accelerate wear and tear, leading to chronic conditions such as tendinitis, carpal tunnel syndrome, and focal dystonia (Berque et al. 2016). Musicians must be responsible and accountable for their health by adopting proper playing techniques to prevent these chronic conditions.

Numerous demographic and physiological factors substantially affect injury risk. Gender disparities suggest that female musicians are more susceptible to playing-related injuries compared to their male counterparts, perhaps attributable to variations in muscle mass, joint flexibility, and hormonal factors (Furuya et al. 2014). Estrogen has been linked to increased ligament laxity, which may contribute to a higher susceptibility to overuse injuries among female musicians (Zaza and Farewell 1997). Instrument choice is another determinant, with string players and pianists exhibiting higher injury rates than wind or brass musicians (Bragge and Murry 2006). This knowledge empowers musicians to be more aware and take necessary precautions to prevent injuries.

Another noteworthy factor is hypermobility, or increased joint flexibility, which is more prevalent among musicians than in the general population (McCormack et al. 2014). While hypermobility may enhance technical ability in some cases, it can also lead to joint instability and increased injury risk. The relationship between hypermobility and playing-related injuries remains inconclusive, with studies presenting mixed findings on whether it is a protective or detrimental factor (Russell et al. 2012). Some research suggests hypermobile musicians experience more significant hand fatigue and discomfort due to reduced joint stability. However, it is reassuring to note that others argue that their adaptability in movement may act as a compensatory advantage in injury prevention (Simmonds and Keer 2007), providing a sense of confidence in the adaptability of hypermobile musicians.

5 Vocal Ergonomics: Challenges and Considerations

Vocal ergonomics is not merely a theoretical concept; it is a fundamental necessity for anyone who relies on their voice professionally. Singers, actors, educators, public speakers, and voice-over artists must recognize that vocal longevity and health are directly linked to the principles of vocal ergonomics, which encompass proper posture, breath control, vocal technique, and overall vocal care. Neglecting these factors can lead to voice disorders, chronic strain, and even irreversible damage to the vocal mechanism, making vocal ergonomics not just an area of academic interest but a critical professional and physiological concern.

5.1 Breath Control and Support

Since breath control directly impacts phonation, resonance, and vocal stamina, it is an essential component of voice production. Vocalists can enhance their vocal performance by practicing effective breath control, particularly diaphragmatic breathing. Vocal fatigue, diminished sound quality, and increased laryngeal tension can all be caused by inadequate air support. According to studies, poor breath control may lead to high subglottic pressure, which raises the risk of injury to the vocal folds (Titze 2000). Singers must learn effective breath management techniques, such as *appoggio* (Italian for "support"), which emphasizes regulated exhalation and the best use of lung capacity to improve breath control and enhance their vocal performance (Sundberg 1993).

5.2 Postural Considerations for Vocal Health

Posture is crucial in vocal health, efficiency, and longevity, particularly for professional voice users such as singers, actors, and teachers. Maintaining an upright, relaxed, and well-aligned posture is essential for optimizing vocal projection, resonance, and breath control. Proper head, neck, spine, and thorax alignment reduces unnecessary strain on the laryngeal muscles, allowing for efficient phonation and unrestricted airflow. Conversely, poor posture, including forward head positioning, excessive muscular tension in the shoulders, or a slouched sitting stance, can negatively impact vocal function by restricting diaphragmatic breathing, reducing breath support, and increasing laryngeal tension (Sapir et al. 1994).

5.2.1 The Impact of Poor Posture on Vocal Function

Postural misalignments contribute to various voice-related dysfunctions, including increased laryngeal strain, reduced vocal endurance, and compromised resonance. Occupational voice research indicates that poor postural habits elevate muscle fatigue, alter phonatory efficiency, and increase the likelihood of vocal injuries (Titze and Verdolini Abbott 2012). For instance, anterior head posture—a common issue in individuals with prolonged screen exposure or desk work—can lead to muscular tension in the neck and shoulders, consequently affecting laryngeal stability and vocal fold vibration. Similarly, slouching reduces the ribcage's expansion capacity, impairing the singer's ability to sustain phrases with adequate breath support. These issues can lead to vocal fatigue, strain, and potential long-term damage if not addressed.

5.2.2 Postural Techniques for Enhancing Vocal Efficiency

Given the significant impact of posture on voice production, voice professionals and pedagogues recommend structured postural training as part of vocal health education. Two widely recognized methodologies that emphasize postural awareness and neuromuscular re-education are as follows:

1. *The Alexander Technique*—This method focuses on reducing excess tension, improving bodily alignment, and enhancing overall coordination to support effortless vocal production. It helps singers and speakers recognize habitual postural imbalances contributing to inefficient voice use (Conable 2000). Studies suggest that integrating Alexander Technique principles into vocal training results in improved breath support, reduced vocal fatigue, and greater vocal clarity (Cacciatore et al. 2011).
2. *The Feldenkrais Method*—A movement-based approach that aims to increase bodily awareness and functional movement patterns through gentle somatic exercises. It is particularly beneficial for minimizing unnecessary muscular tension and facilitating more unrestrained vocal expression. Research highlights its effectiveness in enhancing vocal range, articulation, and overall voice quality by promoting greater adaptability in postural coordination (Mills and Lucchini 2010).

5.2.3 The Role of Educators in Promoting Healthy Postural Habits

Given the critical relationship between posture and vocal health, educators and vocal coaches play a vital role in instilling postural awareness from an early stage. Incorporating body alignment exercises, breath coordination drills, and tension-release techniques into vocal training can help prevent long-term vocal strain and injuries. Additionally, interdisciplinary approaches that integrate physiotherapy, somatic movement therapy, and vocal pedagogy can offer comprehensive strategies for maintaining optimal vocal function throughout a singer's or speaker's career. These approaches can address not only posture and breath control but also the vocal professional's overall physical and mental well-being.

5.3 Avoiding Vocal Strain and Fatigue: Strategies for Sustainable Voice Use

Vocal strain and fatigue are among the most common challenges professional voice users face, including singers, actors, educators, and public speakers. Prolonged vocal use, excessive volume, and improper technique can lead to phonotrauma, characterized by vocal nodules, polyps, and edema (Sataloff 2017). These pathologies result from chronic mechanical stress on the vocal folds, often exacerbated by insufficient vocal rest, poor hydration, and inefficient vocal production techniques. Without proper intervention, repetitive strain can lead to long-term voice disorders, reduced vocal agility, and diminished endurance, ultimately compromising performance and career longevity.

5.3.1 The Physiological Impact of Vocal Strain

Vocal strain occurs when the intrinsic laryngeal muscles—which regulate vocal fold tension and vibration—are subjected to excessive force or prolonged contraction without adequate recovery. This strain can cause microtrauma in the vocal fold tissue, leading to inflammation, stiffness, and impaired phonation (Welham and Maclagan 2003). Over time, the accumulation of these micro-injuries may result in scar tissue formation, reduced vibratory flexibility, and chronic dysphonia.

Several contributing factors accelerate vocal fatigue and strain:

1. *Increased Subglottic Pressure*—Excessive vocal intensity or improper breath support can lead to over-compression of the vocal folds, causing muscle fatigue and phonatory inefficiency.
2. *Tension and Hyperfunction*—Overuse of extrinsic laryngeal muscles, including excessive jaw, tongue, and neck muscle engagement, restricts laryngeal mobility and resonance, contributing to voice fatigue and strain (LeBorgne and Rosenberg 2021).
3. *Phonatory Habits*—Speaking behaviors such as excessive glottal attack, prolonged vocal fry, or compensatory throat tension can increase vocal fold stress and lead to dysphonia and chronic hoarseness (Colton et al. 2011).
4. *Inadequate Recovery*—Just as athletes require rest and conditioning to prevent injury, vocalists must incorporate vocal rest periods to allow the vocal folds to recover from exertion.

5.3.2 Strategies for Minimizing Vocal Strain and Fatigue

To maintain vocal health and longevity, voice users must adopt preventive and rehabilitative techniques that optimize vocal efficiency and reduce strain.

1. *Hydration and Vocal Hygiene*
   - Systemic hydration, or simply drinking enough water, is a powerful tool in your vocal health arsenal. It ensures the vocal fold mucosa remains lubricated, reducing friction and strain (Sivasankar and Leydon 2010).
   - Avoid caffeine, alcohol, and diuretics, contributing to dehydration and increased phonatory effort.

2. *Vocal Warm-Ups and Cool-Downs*
   - Just as physical warm-ups prepare muscles for exertion, vocal warm-ups increase blood circulation, vocal fold flexibility, and resonance efficiency.
   - Gentle phonation exercises such as lip trills, sirens, and humming enhance laryngeal coordination and reduce stiffness before extended use.
   - Cool-down exercises—such as light humming or gentle descending glides—help relax the vocal folds and minimize post-exertion strain (Miller 2008).
3. *Semi-Occluded Vocal Tract Exercises (SOVTE)*
   - Research indicates that SOVTE techniques, such as straw phonation, lip trills, and voiced fricatives, promote efficient vocal fold closure and reduced subglottic pressure (Guzman et al. 2013).
   - These exercises create back pressure, which reduces excessive glottal effort, improves vocal economy, and enhances resonance without strain.
4. *Breath Management and Support*
   - Efficient breath control prevents over-reliance on laryngeal tension for phonation.
   - The *appoggio* technique, a balanced breath support strategy, facilitates consistent airflow regulation, preventing excessive muscular effort in the throat (Sundberg 1993).
   - Avoid shallow breathing patterns that increase laryngeal effort and vocal fatigue.
5. *Postural Alignment and Relaxation Techniques*
   - Maintaining an aligned head-neck-spine posture optimizes laryngeal positioning, breath control, and vocal resonance (Conable 2000).
   - Practices such as the Alexander Technique and Feldenkrais Method promote muscle relaxation, reduce tension, and improve vocal efficiency (Mills and Lucchini 2010).
6. *Vocal Rest and Recovery*
   - Strategic voice breaks are not just a luxury but a necessity to prevent overuse and inflammation of the vocal folds (Sataloff 2017).
   - Avoid speaking over background noise, which leads to involuntary vocal strain and shouting.

5.4 Environmental and Lifestyle Considerations

Physiological and technical factors, external environmental conditions, and lifestyle choices influence vocal health. The interplay of these elements can significantly affect vocal efficiency, longevity, and overall performance capabilities. Addressing these considerations is essential for both professional voice users and individuals who rely on their voice for occupational purposes.

5.4.1 Environmental Factors and Their Impact on Vocal Health

1. *Ambient Humidity and Hydration*
   - Maintaining adequate hydration is critical for optimal vocal function. The vocal folds require a thin layer of mucus for smooth vibration, and dry environments can lead to increased friction, irritation, and potential vocal fatigue (Sivasankar and Leydon 2010).
2. *Air Quality and Pollutant Exposure*
   - Airborne pollutants, allergens, and irritants, including dust, smoke, and industrial chemicals, may induce inflammation of the respiratory tract and vocal folds (Titze 2000).
3. *Acoustic and Performance Conditions*
   - Singing or speaking in environments with poor acoustics or excessive background noise forces voice users to increase their vocal effort, leading to unnecessary strain (Gotaas and Starr 1993).

5.4.2 Lifestyle Factors Affecting Vocal Health

1. *Diet and Hydration*
   - An optimal diet is essential for sustaining vocal health. High-caffeine, alcoholic, and spicy or acidic diets can lead to acid reflux, dehydration, and heightened mucus pro-

duction, all of which adversely impact voice performance (Sataloff 2017).

2. *Sleep and Recovery*
   - Sleep deprivation has been linked to reduced vocal endurance, increased phonatory effort, and diminished overall vocal performance (Hunter and Titze 2009).
3. *Stress and Emotional Well-Being*
   - Psychological stress has a direct impact on vocal production. Increased stress levels can lead to excessive muscular tension in the neck, shoulders, and jaw, affecting phonation and resonance (Sapir et al. 1994).
4. *Vocal Load and Recovery Strategies*
   - Prolonged vocal use without sufficient rest periods can lead to overuse injuries such as nodules, edema, or vocal fatigue (Sataloff 2017).

6 Ergonomics of Wind Instruments: Postural and Physiological Considerations

Playing wind instruments demands a complex interplay of biomechanics, respiratory control, and postural stability. Ergonomic considerations are critical to preventing musculoskeletal strain, optimizing performance efficiency, and ensuring the long-term health of musicians.

6.1 Postural Considerations and Musculoskeletal Health

Correct alignment of the head and neck is crucial for ensuring adequate respiratory control and minimizing strain on the cervical spine. Prolonged forward head posture (FHP) while playing specific wind instruments, particularly those requiring asymmetrical positioning (e.g., flute, saxophone), increases the risk of musculoskeletal discomfort and long-term cervical tension (Kava et al. 2010).

6.2 Upper Limb and Hand Positioning

The fine motor control required for playing wind instruments places significant demand on the wrists, fingers, and forearms. Instruments like the clarinet, oboe, and bassoon require sustained finger flexion, which can contribute to repetitive strain injuries (RSIs) such as tendinitis and carpal tunnel syndrome (Ackermann and Driscoll 2010).

6.3 Torso and Core Stability

Core stability plays a fundamental role in providing support for breath management and overall endurance. Slouched posture, typical in seated wind players, reduces lung capacity and restricts diaphragmatic movement, leading to inefficient breath control (Watson 2009).

6.4 Respiratory Mechanics and Breath Control

6.4.1 Diaphragmatic Breathing and Lung Capacity

Effective breath control is a cornerstone of wind instrument performance. Musicians must develop controlled diaphragmatic breathing to sustain phrases, manage dynamics, and maintain tonal quality (Fiz et al. 2008).

6.4.2 Respiratory Fatigue and Overuse

Wind players are susceptible to respiratory fatigue due to the continuous demand for controlled exhalation. Overuse can lead to hyperventilation syndrome or laryngeal tension (Clift 2012).

6.5 Instrument-Specific Ergonomic Challenges

1. *Flute and Asymmetry Issues*
   - The transverse positioning of the flute requires asymmetrical upper-body engagement, leading to lateral spinal deviation

and potential muscular imbalances (Brandfonbrener 2003).

2. *Clarinet and Saxophone Weight Distribution*
   - Clarinet and saxophone players often experience neck and shoulder tension due to the instrument's weight, mainly when misusing neck straps or harnesses (Kella et al. 2017).
3. *Brass Instrument Stability*
   - Brass players, including trumpet and trombone musicians, require firm embouchure control and upper limb stability (Pascual-Leone et al. 1995).

6.6 Strategies for Injury Prevention and Ergonomic Optimization

1. *Warm-Up and Cool-Down Exercises*
   - Incorporating gentle stretches and breathing exercises before and after playing can enhance flexibility and reduce the risk of overuse injuries.
2. *Ergonomic Instrument Modifications*
   - Adjustable thumb rests, ergonomic key placements, and specialized support devices can enhance comfort and playing efficiency.
3. *Physical Conditioning and Cross-Training*
   - Musicians benefit from cross-training activities such as yoga, Pilates, and strength training to maintain muscular balance and endurance.
4. *Regular Breaks and Practice Pacing*
   - Structured practice routines that include breaks can minimize repetitive strain injuries and mental fatigue.

7 Ergonomics of String Instruments

The violin and guitar are examples of string instruments that need complex motor control, exact posture, and prolonged musculoskeletal involvement. Given the repetitive nature of playing and the physical demands associated with technique, ergonomic considerations are not just about preventing injury but also about optimizing performance.

7.1 Ergonomics of Veena and Sitar Playing

7.1.1 Postural Considerations for Veena and Sitar Players

Both the Veena and Sitar require seated postures that demand stability and balance. However, prolonged playing sessions can contribute to muscle fatigue and postural imbalances due to the weight and size of these instruments.

7.1.1.1 Veena Posture and Challenges

The Veena is traditionally played in a seated position, with the instrument resting on the musician's lap and the large resonator (kudam) placed on the floor. Key ergonomic considerations include the following:

- *Seated Posture*: The musician typically sits cross-legged with the instrument positioned diagonally across the body. This asymmetrical posture can lead to uneven weight distribution, potentially causing lower back strain.
- *Left-Hand Positioning*: The left-hand presses the frets and produces gamakas (ornamental notes), requiring precise finger movements and sustained pressure. Excessive force or improper wrist alignment may contribute to tendinitis and carpal tunnel syndrome (Brandfonbrener 2009b).
- *Right-Hand Movements*: The right hand plucks the strings with a plectrum (mizrab) or fingers. Poor wrist positioning can lead to strain in the forearm muscles, increasing the risk of repetitive strain injuries (RSIs) (Kella et al. 2017).

7.1.1.2 Sitar Posture and Challenges

The Sitar is played semi-cross-legged, with the instrument resting on the musician's left foot, while the resonator (tumba) supports its weight against the body. Ergonomic challenges include the following:

- *Instrument Stability*: Since the Sitar lacks direct body support, musicians often exert pressure with their left leg to stabilize the instrument. This may induce tension in the lower back and hip flexors, particularly during extended performances (Ackermann et al. 2012).
- *Left-Hand Mechanics*: The left hand continuously presses and slides along the frets for meend (gliding notes). This repetitive action can result in hyperextension injuries in the fingers (Horvath 2010).
- *Right-Hand Techniques*: The right-hand uses a plectrum (mizrab) to strike the strings, requiring controlled wrist and finger movement. Excessive wrist flexion or forceful strumming can lead to overuse injuries (Guptill and Zaza 2010).

7.1.2 Biomechanical Challenges in Playing Veena and Sitar

7.1.2.1 Weight Distribution and Spinal Health

The asymmetrical positioning of these instruments can lead to musculoskeletal imbalances:

- *Lower Back Strain*: The one-sided weight distribution of the Veena and Sitar places additional pressure on the spine, leading to discomfort in the lumbar region (Fry 1986).
- *Neck and Shoulder Tension*: Musicians often tilt their heads slightly to maintain visual contact with the frets. Prolonged neck flexion may contribute to cervical spine strain and tension headaches (Chan and Ackermann 2014).

7.1.2.2 Hand and Finger Strain

- *Excessive Finger Pressure*: Prolonged pressure on the strings may result in numbness and discomfort in the fingertips, potentially progressing to problems like trigger finger if left unaddressed.
- *Wrist Deviation*: Unnatural wrist angles while fretting or plucking can increase the risk of carpal tunnel syndrome (Zaza and Farewell 1997).

7.1.2.3 Repetitive Motion Injuries

Prolonged practice sessions without breaks increase the likelihood of developing repetitive motion injuries:

- *Tendonitis*: The repetitive motion of plucking and pressing the strings may lead to inflammation of the tendons in the forearm and wrist (Brandfonbrener 2009b).
- *Bursitis*: Sustained pressure on the left knee due to the instrument's weight (especially in Sitar playing) can cause inflammation in the knee joint (Ackermann and Adams 2004b).

7.1.3 Preventive Strategies for Injury Reduction

7.1.3.1 Postural Adjustments and Supportive Equipment

- *Ergonomic Seating*: A cushioned, slightly elevated seat can help maintain spinal alignment and reduce lower back strain (Guptill and Zaza 2010).
- *Instrument Modifications*: Some musicians use an adjustable footrest or padded support under the Sitar to minimize stress on the left leg (Kella et al. 2017).

7.1.3.2 Hand and Wrist Health

- *Wrist-Neutral Positioning*: Keeping the wrist neutral minimizes tension and reduces strain on the tendons (Zaza 1998).
- *Strength and Flexibility Exercises*: Incorporating hand-stretching exercises and finger-strengthening routines can improve endurance and prevent cramping (Fry 1986).

7.1.3.3 Playing Habits and Workload Management

- *Regular Breaks*: Musicians should follow the 20-20-20 rule—taking a 20 s break every 20 min to stretch and reposition (Ackermann and Adams 2004b).
- *Gradual Increase in Practice Duration*: Sudden increases in practice time elevate the

risk of strain; a structured practice schedule with incremental increases helps in injury prevention (Horvath 2010).

7.2 Ergonomics of Violin Playing

7.2.1 Postural Considerations

The violin is played in an asymmetrical position, requiring stability in the neck, shoulders, and upper limbs. Poor posture can contribute to musculoskeletal strain and performance-related injuries.

- *Neck and Shoulder Alignment*:
  - Violinists hold the instrument between the jaw and shoulder, significantly stressing the cervical spine and shoulder girdle. Prolonged neck rotation and lateral flexion can lead to muscle imbalances and conditions such as cervical dystonia (Schneider and Davidson 2020).
- *Spinal Alignment*:
  - A neutral spine position is essential to prevent kyphotic (hunched) posture. Violinists who maintain an upright stance minimize unnecessary stress on the lower back and improve breathing efficiency for phrasing and endurance (Fry 1986).
- *Arm and Wrist Positioning*:
  - The left hand must maintain an ergonomic position while pressing strings against the fingerboard. Hyperextension or excessive tension in the wrist can lead to tendonitis or carpal tunnel syndrome. Proper bowing technique, with relaxed wrist movements and controlled arm engagement, can prevent forearm fatigue (Rickert et al. 2013).

7.2.2 Common Injuries and Prevention Strategies

7.2.2.1 Neck and Shoulder Strain

- Caused by prolonged tension in the trapezius and sternocleidomastoid muscles.
- *Preventive Measures*: Adjusting shoulder and chin rests, frequent breaks, and targeted stretching (Kella et al. 2017).

7.2.2.2 Wrist and Hand Disorders

- Overusing the left-hand fingers can lead to De Quervain's tenosynovitis (inflammation of tendons in the thumb) (Quarrier 2011).
- *Preventive Measures*: Hand-strengthening exercises, warm-ups, and ensuring natural wrist positioning while shifting or playing in higher positions.

7.2.2.3 Bowing-Related Issues

- Overusing the right shoulder due to repetitive bowing can lead to rotator cuff injuries (Ackermann and Adams 2004b).
- *Preventive Measures*: Balanced bow grip, avoiding excessive force, and using fluid arm movement.

7.2.3 Ergonomic Solutions for Violinists

- *Adjustable Chin and Shoulder Rests*: Customization allows violinists to maintain a natural head and shoulder position.
- *Bow Hold Adjustments*: A relaxed grip prevents excessive strain on the wrist and forearm.
- *Physical Conditioning*: Strengthening the upper back, shoulders, and core helps maintain posture.

7.3 Ergonomics of Guitar Playing

7.3.1 Postural Considerations

Guitarists adopt various playing postures depending on the style (classical, acoustic, electric). Poor posture can lead to back pain, wrist strain, and shoulder discomfort (Farias et al. 2016).

- *Seated Versus Standing Playing Positions*
  - Classical guitarists often use a footstool to raise one leg, tilting the instrument for better ergonomics. However, prolonged asymmetry may cause lower back strain. Alternative solutions include using a guitar support rest instead of a footstool.

- Electric guitarists often hunch forward when standing, leading to kyphotic posture and spinal strain. Using a strap adjusted at a comfortable height prevents excessive wrist flexion and shoulder stress (Dommerholt 2010).
- *Arm and Wrist Positioning*
  - The fretting hand should have a relaxed wrist position to avoid excessive tension. Hyperflexion of the wrist can contribute to nerve compression disorders such as carpal tunnel syndrome.
  - The picking hand should be relaxed to avoid repetitive stress injuries from strumming or fingerpicking. Proper plectrum grip reduces unnecessary thumb and index finger tension.

7.3.2 Common Injuries and Prevention Strategies

7.3.2.1 Tendinitis and Carpal Tunnel Syndrome

- Guitarists frequently develop overuse injuries in the wrist and forearm due to excessive practice.
- *Preventive Measures*: Wrist-neutral positioning, breaks between playing sessions, and forearm flexibility exercises (Zaza 1998).

7.3.2.2 Back and Neck Pain

- Poor seated posture contributes to chronic lower back and neck pain.
- *Preventive Measures*: Lumbar support, ergonomic chair use, and neutral spine maintenance (Farias et al. 2016).

7.3.2.3 Thumb Pain and Overuse Injuries

- Barre chords require intense thumb pressure, leading to thumb tendonitis.
- *Preventive Measures*: Thumb-strengthening exercises and avoiding excessive pressure on the neck of the guitar.

7.3.3 Ergonomic Solutions for Guitarists

- *Guitar Support Rest*: Provides better posture for seated players without causing back asymmetry.
- *Strap Adjustments for Electric Guitarists*: Keeps the instrument at an ergonomic height to avoid wrist overextension.
- *Hand and Finger Conditioning*: Regular stretching and warm-up exercises reduce overuse strain.

8 Ergonomics of Percussion Instruments

8.1 Introduction

Percussion instruments, which include a diverse range of instruments such as the mridangam, tabla, dhol, kanjira, and ghatam in Indian classical music, require precise hand coordination, repetitive striking movements, and controlled muscle exertion. Percussionists are at high risk for playing-related musculoskeletal disorders (PRMDs) due to the physical demands of their playing technique, posture, and repetitive motion (Zaza 1998).

8.1.1 Postural Considerations in Percussion Performance

Seated Versus Standing Playing Positions
Percussion instruments demand significant physical engagement, and the playing position—whether seated or standing—plays a crucial role in determining the musician's comfort, endurance, and risk of musculoskeletal strain.

8.1.1.1 Seated Position (e.g., Mridangam, Tabla, Kanjira, Ghatam)

Traditional Indian percussion instruments like the mridangam, tabla, kanjira, and ghatam are often played in a cross-legged seated posture on the floor. While this position offers stability and allows for a close connection between the instrument and the player, it also presents significant ergonomic challenges:

Lower Back and Hip Strain

- Prolonged sitting in a cross-legged position can result in uneven weight distribution, exacerbating pressure on the lower back and hip joints (Ackermann and Adams 2004b).
- The natural kyphotic curvature of the spine may be exaggerated, leading to excessive lumbar flexion and spinal compression (Horvath 2010).

Knee and Ankle Discomfort

- Static knee flexion in the cross-legged position can result in reduced venous return, leading to numbness and discomfort, particularly in the legs and feet.
- Sitting without adequate cushioning under the ankles may cause direct pressure on the peroneal nerve, leading to discomfort and tingling sensations.

Instrument-Specific Adjustments

- Mridangam players often tilt the instrument slightly towards them, which requires an asymmetric playing posture.
- Tabla players usually place the instrument on a small ring or wooden base, elevating it slightly.
- Ghatam players place the instrument on their lap and strike it with their hands and fingers, leading to high-impact stress on the palm and wrist joints.

Potential Ergonomic Modifications

- Using a small cushion or yoga block to elevate the hips can help maintain a more neutral spine position and reduce lumbar strain.
- Players should frequently shift their position to redistribute weight and improve circulation.

8.1.1.2 Standing Position (e.g., Dhol, Chenda, Djembe, Madal, Khol)

Percussion instruments such as the dhol, chenda, djembe, and khol are traditionally played in a standing position, often involving dynamic movements.

Spinal and Lower Body Strain

- Prolonged standing, especially when carrying a heavily strapped instrument, can increase spinal compression and lead to postural imbalances (Fry 1986).
- Unequal weight distribution, particularly when an instrument is played asymmetrically on one side of the body, can lead to pelvic misalignment and lower back discomfort.

Shoulder and Neck Tension

- Suspended percussion instruments require shoulder straps, which can create uneven pressure on the trapezius and deltoid muscles (Brandfonbrener 2009b).

Impact on Knee and Ankle Stability

- Percussion instruments that require footwork-based playing styles may lead to excessive ankle dorsiflexion and plantarflexion, increasing the risk of ligament strain.

Potential Ergonomic Modifications

- Evenly distributing weight between both legs and consciously engaging core muscles can help maintain balance and reduce back strain.
- Periodic ankle, calf, and hamstring stretches can improve circulation and reduce fatigue from prolonged standing.

8.1.1.3 Upper Body and Arm Positioning in Percussion Performance

Shoulder Engagement and Overuse Risks

- Many percussion instruments require continuous hand movement with elevated arms, particularly in frame drum techniques or significant drum performances.
- Prolonged shoulder abduction can cause rotator cuff fatigue and impingement syndrome (Brandfonbrener 2009b).

Wrist and Hand Mechanics in Percussion Performance

- Tendinitis, carpal tunnel syndrome, and tenosynovitis are all more likely to happen if you bend and straighten your wrist over and over, especially when hitting drumheads hard (Guptill and Zaza 2010).

Potential Ergonomic Modifications

- Using ergonomic wrist supports or periodically shaking out the hands can alleviate tension buildup.
- Implementing hand warm-up routines, including finger stretching, wrist circles, and grip-strengthening exercises, can reduce strain.

8.1.2 Biomechanical Risks in Percussion Playing

8.1.2.1 Repetitive Strain and Impact Injuries in Percussion Performance

Percussionists engage in highly repetitive hand, wrist, and arm movements that generate significant mechanical impact forces.

Hand and Finger Fatigue

- The metacarpal bones and phalanges experience cumulative microtrauma due to continuous percussive impacts, increasing the risk of stress fractures and inflammation of the interphalangeal joints (Chan and Ackermann 2014).

Common Conditions and Symptoms

1. *Metacarpal Stress Fractures*—Small cracks in the bones of the hand due to repeated impact, causing localized pain and swelling.
2. *Tenosynovitis*—Inflammation of the tendon sheath, leading to discomfort, especially when flexing or extending the fingers.
3. *Joint Inflammation (Arthritis-Like Symptoms)*—Chronic irritation of the finger and wrist joints, resulting in stiffness and reduced range of motion.
4. *Nerve Compression Syndromes (e.g., Carpal Tunnel Syndrome)*—Excessive compression of the median nerve, resulting in paresthesia, hypoesthesia, and muscular weakness in the fingers.

Preventive Strategies

- Implementing hand warm-up routines before playing, including wrist rotations, finger stretching, and grip-strengthening exercises.
- Using padded drumsticks or hand wraps to absorb shock and reduce direct impact stress on the fingers and palms.

Palmar Bruising and Soft Tissue Trauma

- Instruments such as the ghatam, kanjira, and djembe require direct hand-to-instrument contact, subjecting the palms to continuous percussive force.

Common Symptoms and Risks

1. *Palmar Bruising*—Darkened, sore patches on the palm due to capillary damage from excessive striking.
2. *Soft Tissue Microtrauma*—Repeated trauma to the connective tissues of the palm, leading to inflammation and potential fibrosis.
3. *Hypersensitivity or Numbness*—Prolonged exposure to impact stress may result in nerve compression or loss of tactile sensitivity.

Preventive Strategies

- Utilizing hand conditioning techniques to gradually increase tissue resilience and tolerance to impact.
- Incorporating post-performance hand massages and contrast baths to promote circulation and reduce inflammation.

8.1.2.2 Asymmetry and Postural Imbalance in Percussion Performance

Due to the nature of traditional playing styles, percussionists often develop muscular asymmetries, postural imbalances, and spinal misalignments.

One-Sided Playing Pressure and Muscular Asymmetry

- Traditional Indian percussion instruments such as the mridangam, tabla, and pakhawaj involve distinct roles for each hand—one playing higher-pitched strokes while the other producing bass tones (Horvath 2010).

Common Conditions and Symptoms

1. *Tendon Overload and Strain in the Dominant Hand*—Increased likelihood of extensor tendinitis due to continuous fast-paced playing patterns.
2. *Forearm Imbalance*—Unequal muscle development in the flexors and extensors, leading to reduced joint stability and coordination difficulties.

3. *Shoulder and Upper Back Misalignment*—Habitual one-sided playing can cause trapezius overuse and latissimus dorsi tightness, contributing to postural deviation.

Preventive Strategies
- Engaging in bilateral hand coordination exercises to equalize muscle workload and develop symmetrical motor skills.
- Performing cross-training techniques, such as switching dominant hand roles during practice, to reduce unilateral strain.

Leg and Spine Strain from Prolonged Sitting
- Cross-legged seating, as traditionally used for the mridangam, tabla, kanjira, and ghatam, places asymmetric pressure on the legs and lower back (Zaza and Farewell 1997).

Common Conditions and Symptoms
1. *Knee Stiffness and Circulatory Issues*—Reduced blood flow due to prolonged knee flexion, leading to numbness and cramping.
2. *Lower Back Pain and Lumbar Disc Strain*—Excessive forward bending places undue stress on the lumbar vertebrae, increasing the risk of disc herniation and chronic back pain.
3. *Pelvic and Hip Imbalance*—Uneven weight distribution across the hip joints can cause hip flexor tightness and sacral misalignment.

Preventive Strategies
- Use a small cushion or raised support to elevate the hips and maintain a neutral spinal position while seated.
- Alternating between cross-legged and kneeling postures to redistribute pressure and enhance circulation.

8.1.3 Preventive Strategies for Injury Reduction

8.1.3.1 Postural Adjustments and Supportive Equipment

Proper posture and ergonomic support are essential for minimizing physical strain and preventing musculoskeletal issues in musicians playing string instruments such as the Veena, Sitar, Sarod, and Tanpura.

Ergonomic Seating for Spinal Health
- A slightly elevated cushioned seat or ergonomic chair can aid in maintaining spinal alignment and reducing lower back strain, particularly for musicians who perform for extended durations (Guptill and Zaza 2010).

Instrument Modifications and Positional Supports
- Some musicians use an adjustable footrest to elevate one leg slightly, redistributing body weight more evenly and reducing pressure on the spine (Kella et al. 2017).

Preventive Strategies
- Use cushioned support or a low stool to maintain hip and knee comfort.
- Position the instrument to avoid excessive forward bending.

8.1.3.2 Hand and Wrist Health

Musicians playing plucked and fretted string instruments engage in complex finger movements, requiring sustained grip strength, wrist dexterity, and hand endurance.

Wrist-Neutral Positioning for Injury Prevention
- Keeping the wrist in a neutral position reduces tendon tension and lowers the risk of carpal tunnel syndrome (Zaza 1998).

Strength and Flexibility Exercises for Endurance
- Hand-stretching exercises and finger-strengthening routines improve dexterity and reduce the risk of muscle fatigue (Fry 1986).

Preventive Strategies
- Maintain a relaxed grip to prevent overuse injuries.
- Incorporate finger and wrist warm-up exercises before playing.

8.1.3.3 Playing Habits and Workload Management

Maintaining healthy playing habits and managing practice workloads is crucial for preventing musculoskeletal injuries.

Regular Breaks to Reduce Fatigue

- Musicians should follow the 20-20-20 rule—taking a 20 s break every 20 min to stretch, relax the hands, and adjust posture (Ackermann and Adams 2004b).

Gradual Increase in Practice Duration for Injury Prevention

- Sudden increases in playing time or intensity elevate the risk of tendonitis, muscle strain, and repetitive stress injuries (Horvath 2010).

Preventive Strategies

- Avoid sudden increases in practice duration to prevent overuse injuries.
- Implement dynamic stretching before and after playing.

9 Ergonomics of Keyboard Instruments

9.1 Postural Considerations for Keyboard Players

9.1.1 Seated Position and Spinal Alignment

Proper seated posture is fundamental for reducing musculoskeletal strain, improving endurance, and enhancing technical efficiency while playing a keyboard instrument.

Chair Height and Distance

The height of the chair significantly influences postural stability and spinal alignment. The ideal chair height should enable the player to maintain:

- Knees and hips ensure balanced weight distribution at a 90° angle (Horvath 2010).
- Flat foot placement on the floor or a slight footrest prevents excessive hip flexion and reduces lower back tension (Guptill and Zaza 2010).

Feet Placement

Proper foot placement ensures the following:

- Flat foot contact with the ground allows for better spinal support and reduces pelvic tilt.
- A slight forward tilt of the pelvis helps align the spine naturally, preventing excessive lower back curvature.

Back Support and Postural Stability

Long hours of practice without proper back support can lead to lumbar strain, slouching, and fatigue. Maintaining spinal neutrality helps:

- Avoid excessive forward bending, which strains the thoracic and lumbar spine (Fry 1986).

Preventive Strategies

- Use an adjustable, cushioned bench with lumbar support.
- Preserve a neutral spinal alignment and refrain from excessive front bending.

9.1.2 Arm and Wrist Positioning

The arms and wrists are crucial in executing smooth and controlled keystrokes.

Elbow Position

- The elbows should be slightly above or level with the keyboard to allow natural wrist movement without excessive bending (Zaza 1998).

Wrist Alignment

- The wrists should be kept in a neutral position—neither flexed downward nor extended upward—to minimize strain on tendons and nerves (Brandfonbrener 2009b).

Finger Curvature and Hand Positioning

- The fingers should maintain a relaxed, slightly curved position, with minimal hyperextension at the knuckles (Ackermann and Adams 2004b).

Preventive Strategies

- Keep wrists aligned with forearms to avoid excessive flexion.
- Relax your fingers and avoid excess force when pressing keys.

9.2 Common Musculoskeletal Risks and Injury Prevention

9.2.1 Repetitive Strain Injuries (RSIs) in Keyboard Players

Repetitive strain injuries (RSIs) are common among keyboard musicians due to prolonged playing sessions, repetitive hand and finger movements, and static postures.

Carpal Tunnel Syndrome

- Symptoms encompass numbness, tingling, and weakening in the fingers and hand, specifically impacting the thumb, index, and middle fingers (Zaza and Farewell 1997).

Tendinitis and Tenosynovitis

- Symptoms include pain, swelling, and difficulty in finger movement, particularly in high-intensity playing styles (Chan and Ackermann 2014).

Thoracic Outlet Syndrome

- Tingling, weakness, and arm fatigue result from restricted blood flow and nerve compression (Horvath 2010).

Preventive Strategies

- Incorporate frequent micro-breaks to reduce cumulative muscle fatigue.
- Warm-up exercises should be performed before intense playing sessions to increase blood circulation.

9.2.2 Postural Imbalances and Back Strain

Keyboard musicians often spend extended hours in static postures, which may contribute to postural imbalances and chronic musculoskeletal strain.

Forward Head Posture (FHP)

- Leaning forward to read sheet music or look at the keyboard can cause forward head posture (FHP), which puts excess strain on the neck and upper back (Ackermann and Adams 2004b).

Rounded Shoulders and Pectoral Tightness

- Shoulder protraction (hunching forward) results in a weakened upper back and restricted arm movement (Brandfonbrener 2009b).

Lower Back Pain and Lumbar Strain

- Prolonged sitting without adequate lumbar support may cause lower back pain and spinal misalignment (Horvath 2010).

Preventive Strategies

- Maintain an upright, relaxed posture, keeping the shoulders slightly back to avoid tension.
- Use a music stand at eye level to prevent excessive neck flexion and forward head posture.

9.3 Ergonomic Techniques for Injury Prevention

9.3.1 Optimal Keyboard Height and Bench Adjustments

Achieving the correct keyboard height and bench adjustments is crucial for reducing strain on the upper body.

Keyboard Height and Forearm Positioning

- The height of the keyboard should allow the forearms to remain parallel to the floor, preventing excessive flexion or extension of the wrists (Fry 1986).

Adjustable Bench and Seating Position

- The bench should allow for a 90° knee and hip angle, ensuring that the feet remain flat on the floor for stability (Guptill and Zaza 2010).

Hand Placement and Finger Positioning

- Fingers should be slightly curved, preventing hyperextension and unnecessary muscle tension (Horvath 2010).

Preventive Strategies

- Adjust the keyboard height to keep elbows at a comfortable angle, preventing wrist strain.
- Use an adjustable bench to ensure proper spinal and lower body alignment.

9.3.2 Hand and Wrist Exercises for Flexibility and Strength

Regular hand and wrist exercises enhance endurance, prevent stiffness, and minimize injury risks.

Finger Dexterity Drills

- Hanon finger exercises and Czerny's studies effectively build finger strength and agility (Zaza 1998).

Stretching Exercises for Wrist and Hand Mobility

- Wrist flexor and extensor stretches improve the range of motion and prevent conditions like tenosynovitis (Brandfonbrener 2009b).

Foam Ball and Grip-Strengthening Exercises

- Foam ball squeezes strengthen the intrinsic hand muscles, allowing for better finger control (Fry 1986).

Preventive Strategies

- Stretch wrists and fingers before and after playing to maintain flexibility.
- Use foam ball exercises to strengthen intrinsic hand muscles for better control.

9.4 Workload Management and Playing Habits

Proper workload management and structured practice routines are essential for maintaining optimal playing efficiency.

Gradual Increase in Playing Time

- Sudden increases in practice duration place excessive strain on the fingers, wrists, and forearms, heightening the risk of conditions like tendinitis and carpal tunnel syndrome (Horvath 2010).

Frequent Rest Intervals

- The 50-10 rule (50 min of practice followed by 10 min of rest) helps reduce fatigue and stiffness, promoting better muscle recovery and focus (Ackermann and Adams 2004b).

Alternating Between Practice Techniques

- Rotating between different practice techniques ensures balanced muscle engagement, preventing repetitive strain on specific muscle groups.

Preventive Strategies

- Implement the 50-10 rule for structured rest intervals.
- Balance technical exercises with expressive playing to prevent repetitive strain.

10 The Role of Ergonomics in Music Education

Music education traditionally emphasizes technique, musicality, and repertoire development. However, integrating ergonomics into the curriculum is equally vital (Guptill and Zaza 2010).

10.1 Understanding the Physical Demands of Instrumental Performance

Different instruments require specific postures and movements, making ergonomic considerations unique to each musician.

- *Keyboardists*: Maintain neutral wrist alignment to prevent carpal tunnel syndrome (Zaza 1998).
- *String Players*: Proper bowing mechanics and left-hand positioning minimize tension (Horvath 2010).
- *Wind & Brass Players*: Breath support and posture affect tonal consistency (Ackermann and Adams 2004b).
- *Percussionists*: Controlled wrist and arm movements reduce repetitive strain injuries (Chan and Ackermann 2014).

10.2 Incorporating Ergonomics into Practice Sessions

Structured practice routines integrating ergonomic awareness help musicians develop sustainable habits.

10.2.1 Warm-Up and Cool-Down Routines

- Warm-up exercises enhance blood circulation and flexibility, preparing muscles for performance (Guptill and Zaza 2010).

10.2.2 Alternating Practice Techniques

- Repetitive technical drills can lead to overuse injuries. Alternating between technical exercises and expressive playing allows muscles to rest and recover (Brandfonbrener 2009b).

10.3 The Use of Assistive Devices for Ergonomic Support

Integrating ergonomic accessories and instrument modifications enhances comfort and reduces the risk of musculoskeletal strain.

10.3.1 Seating and Instrument Support

- Adjustable chairs with lumbar support promote spinal alignment (Ackermann and Adams 2004b).

10.3.2 Hand and Wrist Support

- Wrist supports and ergonomic keyboard stands help maintain neutral hand positioning (Fry 1986).

10.4 Educating Musicians on Long-Term Health and Injury Prevention

Incorporating injury prevention into music curricula equips students with lifelong skills for maintaining physical well-being.

10.4.1 Integrating Ergonomics into Music Pedagogy

- Schools and conservatories should offer courses on musicians' health and wellness (Horvath 2010).

10.4.2 Encouraging Self-Assessment and Awareness

- Regular self-assessment helps musicians recognize early signs of tension or discomfort (Brandfonbrener 2009b).

11 Conclusion

Integrating ergonomics into a musician's practice and education is not just a necessity, but a powerful tool for taking control of one's long-term physical health, technical proficiency, and artistic expression. Playing an instrument requires dexterity, stamina, and repetitive motions, all of which can adversely affect the body. Nonetheless, musicians can considerably lower their risk of musculoskeletal conditions, repetitive strain injuries, and postural imbalances by practicing good ergonomic awareness (Guptill and Zaza 2010).

A structured approach to ergonomics encompasses multiple aspects, including posture optimization, body mechanics, structured practice routines, and the use of assistive devices. Proper posture ensures musicians maintain spinal alignment, minimize muscular tension, and reduce unnecessary strain on joints. Effective body mechanics like relaxed hand positioning and fluid movement transitions allow for greater technical precision and endurance. Additionally, structured practice routines incorporating regular breaks, warm-up and cool-down exercises, and variation in playing techniques help mitigate the risk of overuse injuries (Ackermann and Adams 2004b).

Incorporating ergonomic principles into music education fosters a culture of injury prevention and long-term wellness. Early awareness of movement efficiency, breath control, and postural alignment allows musicians to build sustainable habits from the outset of their training. By integrating disciplines such as the Alexander Technique, Feldenkrais Method, and yoga, musicians can better understand their biomechanics and learn to identify and correct harmful playing patterns (Mills and Lucchini 2010).

A musician's ability to maintain peak performance and artistic excellence is intrinsically tied to their physical well-being. Musicians can cultivate a sustainable career free from debilitating injuries by continuously assessing their playing techniques and adapting them to ensure ergonomic efficiency (Horvath 2010).

References

Ackermann B, Adams R (2004a) Perceptions of pain and injury among string players. Med Probl Perform Art 19(2):56–64

Ackermann B, Adams R (2004b) Physical characteristics and pain patterns of skilled violinists. Med Probl Perform Art 19(2):65–71

Ackermann B, Driscoll T (2010) Development of a new instrument for musicians' health: the musicians' health and wellness survey. Med Probl Perform Art 25(4):147–155

Ackermann B, Driscoll T, Kenny DT (2012) Musculoskeletal pain and injury in professional orchestral musicians in Australia. Med Probl Perform Art 27(4):181–187

Baadjou VA, Roussel NA, Verbunt JA, Smeets RJ, de Bie RA (2016) Systematic review: risk factors for musculoskeletal disorders in musicians. Occup Med 66(8):614–622

Berque P, Gray H, McFadyen A (2016) Playing-related musculoskeletal problems in professional musicians: a longitudinal cohort study. Med Probl Perform Art 31(1):1–8

Bragge P, Murry S (2006) Vocal health and pedagogy: science and application, vol 1. Plural Publishing, San Diego

Brandfonbrener AG (2003) Musculoskeletal problems of wind instrumentalists. Med Probl Perform Art 18(2):57–63

Brandfonbrener AG (2009a) Musicians and the prevention of injury. Occup Med 59(6):390–396

Brandfonbrener AG (2009b) Musculoskeletal problems of instrumental musicians. Hand Clin 25(1):101–111

Cacciatore TW, Gurfinkel VS, Horak FB, Day BL (2011) Prolonged weight-shift and altered spinal coordination during sit-to-stand in practitioners of the Alexander Technique. Gait Posture 34(4):496–501

Chan C, Ackermann B (2014) Evidence-informed physical therapy management of performance-related musculoskeletal disorders in musicians. Front Psychol 5:706

Clift S (2012) Singing, wellbeing, and health. In: MacDonald R, Kreutz G, Mitchell L (eds) Music, health, and wellbeing. Oxford University Press, Oxford, pp 113–124

Colton RH, Casper JK, Leonard R (2011) Understanding voice problems: a physiological perspective for diagnosis and treatment, 4th edn. Lippincott Williams & Wilkins, Baltimore

Conable B (2000) What every singer needs to know about the body. GIA Publications, Chicago

Dommerholt J (2010) Playing-related pain problems in guitarists. Med Probl Perform Art 25(4):187–195

Farias G, Brum P, Freitas FS (2016) Postural risk factors for guitarists: a biomechanical and physiological analysis. J Bodyw Mov Ther 20(1):123–130

Fiz JA, Romero J, Conejero J, Llatas M, Izquierdo M (2008) Respiratory muscle training in wind musicians: effects on pulmonary function and performance. J Voice 22(6):683–689

Fry HJH (1986) Overuse syndrome in musicians: prevention and management. Lancet 328(8509):728–731

Furuya S, Nakahara H, Aoki T, Kinoshita H (2014) Prevalence and causal factors of playing-related musculoskeletal disorders in instrumental musicians. Med Probl Perform Art 29(4):198–204

Gotaas C, Starr A (1993) Vocal fatigue among teachers. J Voice 7(4):339–344

Guptill CA, Zaza C (2010) Injury prevention: what music teachers can do. Music Educ J 96(4):28–34

Guzman M, Finizia C, Lindestad P-Å, Larsson H (2013) Vocal tract and glottal function during and after vocal warm-up: high-speed videoendoscopy and spectral analysis. J Voice 27(5):674.e1–674.e10. Available at: https://doi.org/10.1016/j.jvoice.2013.03.005

Horvath J (2010) Playing (less) hurt: an injury prevention guide for musicians. Hal Leonard Corporation, Milwaukee

Hunter EJ, Titze IR (2009) Variability in vocal outcomes due to dehydration and vocal load. J Speech Lang Hear Res 52(4):822–835

Kava KS, Larson CA, Stiller CH (2010) Postural analysis of wind instrument players. Med Probl Perform Art 25(3):115–120

Kella K, Chong J, Hough DG (2017) Effects of ergonomic interventions on string instrument musicians. J Occup Rehabil 27(2):421–431

LeBorgne WD, Rosenberg M (2021) The vocal athlete, 2nd edn. Plural Publishing, San Diego

McCormack M, Briggs J, Hakim AJ (2014) Joint hypermobility and musculoskeletal injuries in musicians. Med Probl Perform Art 29(3):143–148

Miller R (2008) Solutions for singers: tools for performers and teachers. Oxford University Press, New York

Mills C, Lucchini L (2010) Postural alignment and vocal efficiency: the role of the Alexander Technique in vocal training. J Sing 67(3):345–360

Paarup HM, Baelum J, Holm JW, Manniche C, Wedderkopp N (2011) Prevalence and consequences of musculoskeletal symptoms in symphony orchestra musicians vary by gender: a cross-sectional study. BMC Musculoskelet Disord 12:223

Pascual-Leone A, Nguyet D, Cohen LG, Brasil-Neto JP, Cammarota A, Hallett M (1995) Modulation of muscle responses evoked by transcranial magnetic stimulation during the acquisition of new fine motor skills. J Neurophysiol 74(3):1037–1045

Quarrier N (2011) Performing arts medicine: assessing and treating the instrumental musician. Phys Med Rehabil Clin 22(3):553–566

Ranelli S, Straker L, Smith A (2014) Playing-related musculoskeletal problems in children learning instrumental music: the association with age, gender, and music exposure factors. Med Probl Perform Art 29(2):75–81

Rickert DL, Barrett J, Ackermann B (2013) A study of right arm and bowing technique among violinists. Med Probl Perform Art 28(2):65–71

Russell JA, Shave RM, Yoshioka M (2012) Hypermobility and its implications for musicians' health. Med Probl Perform Art 27(4):203–209

Sapir S, Mathers-Schmidt K, Larson DL (1994) Vocal fatigue in teachers: a review of vocal load and vocal endurance. J Voice 8(2):79–84

Sataloff RT (2017) Vocal health and pedagogy: advanced assessment and practice, 2nd edn. Plural Publishing, San Diego

Schneider E, Davidson J (2020) Physical demands and postural adaptations in violin playing. Music Med 12(3):144–151

Simmonds JV, Keer RJ (2007) Hypermobility and the hypermobility syndrome. Man Ther 12(4):298–309

Sivasankar MP, Leydon C (2010) The role of hydration in vocal fold physiology. Laryngoscope 120(1):153–158

Sundberg J (1993) The science of the singing voice. Northern Illinois University Press, DeKalb

Titze IR (2000) Principles of voice production. National Center for Voice and Speech, Iowa City

Titze IR, Verdolini Abbott K (2012) Vocology: the science and practice of voice habilitation. National Center for Voice and Speech, Salt Lake City

Watson AHD (2009) The biology of musical performance and performance-related injury. Scarecrow Press, Lanham

Welham NV, Maclagan MA (2003) Vocal fold histopathology associated with heavy vocal load: a review. J Voice 17(4):509–518. Available at: https://doi.org/10.1016/S0892-1997(03)00046-6

Zaza C (1998) Playing-related musculoskeletal disorders in musicians: a systematic review of incidence and prevalence. Can Med Assoc J 158(8):1019–1025

Zaza C, Farewell VT (1997) Musicians' playing-related musculoskeletal disorders: an examination of risk factors. Am J Ind Med 32(3):292–300

Performance-Related Musculoskeletal Disorders in Musicians: An Integrated Orthopaedic and Radiological Perspective

Karthikeyan P. Iyengar, Veenadhari Bhamidipaty, and Rajesh Botchu

Contents

K. P. Iyengar
Department of Orthopaedics, Southport and Ormskirk Hospitals, Mersey and West Lancashire NHS Trust, Southport, UK

V. Bhamidipaty
Department of CSE, GITAM, Visakhapatnam, India

R. Botchu (✉)
Department of MSK Radiology, Royal Orthopaedic Hospital, Birmingham, UK

Med Radiol Diagn Imaging (2025)

https://doi.org/10.1007/174_2025_630,

Published Online: 26 October 2025

Abstract

Instrumental musicians, whether performing in Western orchestras or Indian classical traditions, face a high risk of performance-related musculoskeletal disorders (PRMDs), which manifest as pain, weakness, numbness, or tingling that impair their ability to play at their accustomed level. With a lifetime prevalence of 60%–90%, PRMDs result from repetitive motions, awkward postures, forceful exertions, and, occasionally, vibration inherent to specific instruments. This chapter integrates orthopaedic principles—encompassing epidemiology, biomechanics, diagnostics, management, and prevention—with radiological insights to enhance diagnostic precision through advanced imaging modalities like MRI, ultrasound, and X-ray. It emphasizes instrument-specific stressors, particularly those affecting Indian classical musicians who adopt cross-legged or kneeling postures, which pose unique biomechanical challenges. Clinicians diagnose PRMDs using detailed, instrument-specific history, thorough physical examinations, and targeted imaging to identify underlying pathologies. They prioritize conservative management, including physiotherapy, ergonomic retraining, and activity modification, reserving surgical interventions for severe or refractory cases. Emerging technologies, such as wearable sensors, support preventive strategies to ensure sustainable musical careers. This multidisciplinary approach equips clinicians with a robust framework to manage PRMDs effectively, safeguarding musicians' health and professional longevity.

1 Introduction

Instrumental musicians, whether mastering a violin in a symphony orchestra or a sitar in a raga performance, dedicate extraordinary physical and mental effort to their craft. This commitment, however, often triggers performance-related musculoskeletal disorders (PRMDs), which cause pain, weakness, numbness, or tingling, hindering peak performance (Zaza et al. 1998). Unlike acute sports injuries, PRMDs develop from cumulative microtrauma due to repetitive motions, sustained awkward postures, and forceful exertions tailored to each instrument's demands. Indian classical musicians face additional biomechanical stressors from traditional cross-legged or kneeling postures, particularly affecting the spine, hips, and knees.

Orthopaedic specialists analyse the biomechanical origins of PRMDs, diagnose through meticulous physical examinations, and manage with rehabilitation strategies customized to the musician's instrument and practice habits. Radiologists enhance this approach by visualizing soft tissue, joint, and nerve pathologies using imaging modalities like magnetic resonance imaging (MRI), ultrasound, X-ray, and computed tomography (CT). These tools reveal the structural consequences of biomechanical stress, enabling precise diagnosis and guiding treatment plans.

This chapter synthesizes orthopaedic and radiological expertise to provide clinicians in performing arts medicine with a comprehensive resource. It examines PRMD epidemiology and prevalence, identifies instrument-specific biomechanical stressors, classifies injury mechanisms, and outlines diagnostic and management strategies. It highlights the unique challenges Indian classical musicians face due to traditional playing postures that heighten specific musculoskeletal risks. By combining clinical examination with advanced imaging, this chapter equips healthcare professionals to diagnose, treat, and prevent PRMDs, ensuring musicians sustain their careers without compromising their health.

2 Epidemiology and Prevalence

Epidemiological studies report that instrumental musicians experience a lifetime PRMD prevalence of 60%–90% (Zaza 1998; Baadjou et al. 2016). Professional orchestral musicians face a particularly high burden, with 12-month prevalence rates ranging from 41% to 93% (Silva et al. 2015). A study of 243 British symphony orchestra members revealed that 86% experienced musculoskeletal pain in the past year, with over 80% reporting symptoms severe enough to impair performance (Leaver et al. 2011). Conservatory students also suffer, with 30%–50% reporting PRMDs, indicating early onset during musical training (Yoshimura et al. 2008; Roach et al. 1994).

Indian classical musicians face similar challenges. A study of 96 dhol players found that 96.9% reported pain over 12 months, with 67.7% experiencing low back pain and 54.2% reporting shoulder pain (Chandran et al. 2022). Another study of 35 Indian classical instrumentalists noted that 91% suffered wrist or hand pain, and 89% reported low back pain, underscoring the impact of cross-legged postures (Mishra et al. 2013).

Certain factors heighten PRMD risk. String players, such as violinists, violists, and sitarists, report the highest prevalence (67%) compared to wind players (54%) or percussionists, who benefit from varied postures (Davies and Mangion 2002; Fotiadis et al. 2013). Female musicians face a 70% prevalence compared to 52% in men, possibly due to differences in muscle mass, joint laxity, or hormonal effects on connective tissues (Paarup et al. 2011). Older musicians (50–61 years) report a 91% prevalence, compared to 83% in younger musicians (22–29 years), likely due to cumulative degenerative changes (Zetterberg et al. 1998).

These findings highlight the need for targeted diagnostics, including advanced imaging, to identify specific PRMD pathologies. Clinicians prioritize high-risk groups—such as string players, female musicians, and Indian classical performers—for early intervention and prevention.

3 Biomechanical Analysis and Instrument-Specific Stressors

PRMDs stem from biomechanical stressors—repetitive motion, awkward postures, forceful exertion, and occasional vibration—that differ by instrument group. Radiologists use imaging to visualize the structural consequences of these stressors, from muscle oedema to tendon tears and nerve compression. This section analyses biomechanical challenges and corresponding pathologies for major instrument groups, with imaging findings guiding diagnosis.

3.1 String Instruments (Table 1) (e.g. Violin, Sitar, Sarod, Guitar)

String instrument players adopt asymmetric postures that strain the musculoskeletal system. Violinists and violists maintain static shoulder elevation and neck tilting to support their instruments, causing cervical strain, trapezius myalgia, rotator cuff tendinopathy, and lateral epicondylitis (Ackermann and Adams 2003). Indian classical musicians, such as sitarists and sarod players, sit cross-legged, stressing the hips and lower back and increasing risks of lumbar strain and hip impingement (Mishra et al. 2013). Guitarists face similar risks from repetitive wrist and finger motions.

Radiologists rely on MRI to detect soft tissue changes, such as muscle oedema in cervical strain or partial rotator cuff tears. Ultrasound

Table 1 Imaging findings for string instrument-related pathologies

Pathology	Imaging modality	Key findings
Cervical strain	MRI	Muscle oedema, subtle disc bulges
Trapezius myalgia	MRI	Muscle hypertrophy or oedema (if pathological)
Rotator cuff tendinopathy	MRI	Tendinosis, bursitis, partial tears (e.g. supraspinatus)
Rotator cuff tendinopathy	Ultrasound	Tendon hyperaemia, fluid, thickening
Lateral epicondylitis (Figs. 5 and 6)	MRI	Partial-thickness tears of extensor tendons, oedema at lateral epicondyle
Lateral epicondylitis (Fig. 7)	Ultrasound	Hypoechoic tendons, increased vascularity

provides dynamic assessment of tendon hyperaemia and thickening, particularly in lateral epicondylitis.

3.2 Woodwind and Brass Instruments (Table 2) (e.g. Bansuri, Shehnai, Nadaswaram)

Woodwind and brass players maintain forward head postures and protracted shoulders to support their instruments, often sitting cross-legged in Indian traditions. These positions cause neck pain, tension headaches, temporomandibular joint (TMJ) stress, and shoulder impingement (Kaufman-Cohen and Ratzon 2011). The sustained embouchure required for blowing instruments strains cervical muscles and the jaw, contributing to degenerative changes and joint effusion.

Radiologists use MRI to confirm degenerated cervical discs and facet arthropathy in neck pain, while CT detects osteophytes in TMJ stress. Ultrasound assesses shoulder impingement, identifying rotator cuff bursitis and dynamic compression.

Table 2 Imaging findings for woodwind and brass instrument-related pathologies

Pathology	Imaging modality	Key findings
Neck pain (cervical degeneration)	MRI	Degenerated discs, facet arthropathy, disc bulges
Neck pain (cervical degeneration)	X-ray	Abnormal lordosis or kyphosis
Tension headaches	MRI	Cervical muscle strain, subtle disc issues
TMJ stress	MRI/CT	Osteophytes, joint effusion
Shoulder strain (impingement)	MRI/ ultrasound	Rotator cuff impingement, bursitis

Table 3 Imaging findings for percussion instrument-related pathologies

Pathology	Imaging modality	Key findings
Low back pain (lumbar degeneration)	MRI	Disc bulges, Modic changes, loss of lordosis
Low back pain (lumbar degeneration)	X-ray	Spondylotic changes, osteophytes
Hip labral rears	MRI arthrography	Labral fraying, femoroacetabular impingement
Knee meniscal tears (Fig. 1)	MRI	Meniscal tears, chondromalacia, pes anserine bursitis

3.3 Percussion Instruments (Table 3) (e.g. Tabla, Mridangam, Dhol)

Percussionists, particularly in Indian classical music, adopt kneeling or cross-legged postures that load the hips, knees, and lower back. These positions, combined with repetitive striking motions, cause low back pain, lumbar disc degeneration, hip labral tears, and knee meniscal tears (Chandran et al. 2022). The forceful nature of percussion playing heightens shoulder and elbow tendinitis risks.

Radiologists use MRI to detect disc bulges and Modic changes in lumbar degeneration, while X-rays reveal spondylotic changes. MRI arthrography identifies hip labral tears, and standard MRI confirms knee meniscal tears and chondromalacia.

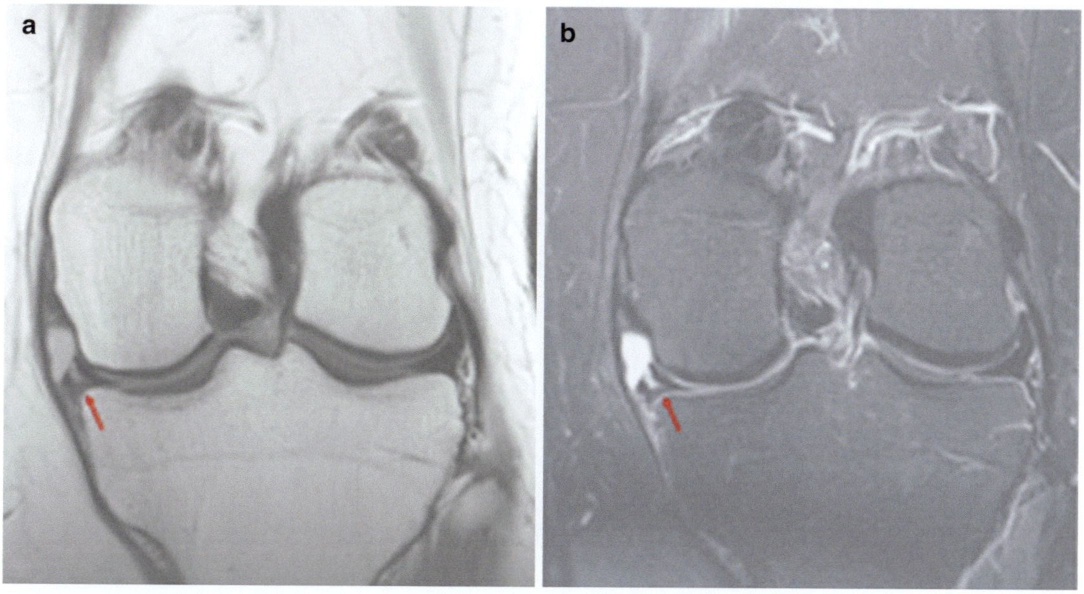

Fig. 1 Coronal PD (**a**) and PDFS (**b**) show medial meniscal tear with parameniscal cyst (arrow)

3.4 Keyboard Instruments (Table 4) (e.g. Piano, Harmonium)

Keyboardists, whether playing a piano or harmonium, lean forward and perform repetitive wrist and finger motions, often while seated cross-legged in Indian traditions. These postures cause lumbar strain, neck and upper back pain, and wrist tendonitis, including trigger finger and De Quervain's tenosynovitis (Fig. 2) (Bragge et al. 2006). The sustained forward posture exacerbates cervical and lumbar stress, while repetitive hand movements heighten nerve entrapment risks.

Radiologists use MRI and X-ray to detect degenerative spinal changes, while ultrasound visualizes tendon thickening and fluid accumulation in wrist tendonitis.

Table 4 Imaging findings for keyboard instrument-related pathologies

Pathology	Imaging modality	Key findings
Lumbar strain	MRI/X-ray	Mild degenerative changes, postural kyphosis
Neck/upper back pain	MRI	Cervical disc bulges, muscle oedema
Wrist tendonitis (Fig. 3)	Ultrasound	Tendon thickening, fluid (e.g. trigger finger)

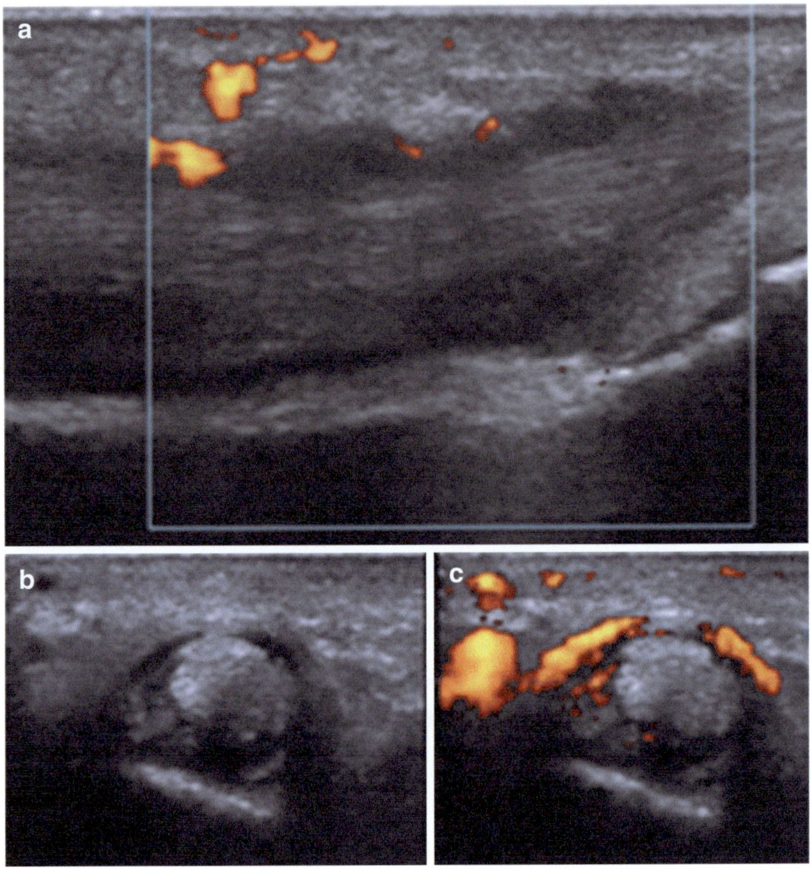

Fig. 2 Longitudinal with Doppler (**a**), short axis (**b**), and colour Doppler (**c**) showing marked flexor tenosynovitis with increased signal on Doppler

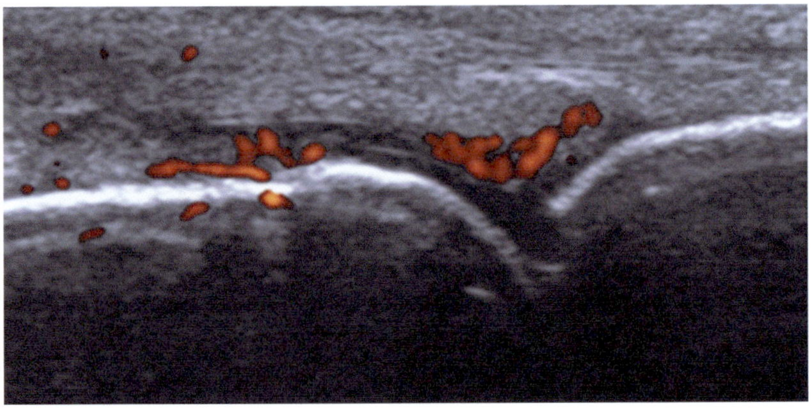

Fig. 3 Longitudinal ultrasound of the MCPJ (metacarpophalangeal joint) of the index finger shows small effusion with synovitis and marked increased signal on Doppler

4 Classification and Mechanisms of Injury

Clinicians classify PRMDs based on their underlying mechanisms, with radiologists using imaging to provide diagnostic clarity. The following categories outline the primary injury types in musicians, each with distinct biomechanical triggers and imaging findings:

- *Muscle/Tendon Overuse* (Table 5): Repetitive microtrauma causes tendinitis or tendinosis, such as supraspinatus tendinitis in violinists, accounting for 76.6% of orchestral PRMDs (Steinmetz et al. 2015). Radiologists use MRI to reveal tendinosis or partial tears, while ultrasound shows thickened tendons with hyperaemia.
- *Nerve Entrapment Syndromes* (Table 6): Compression syndromes, such as carpal tunnel syndrome (CTS) in pianists or ulnar neuropathy in flutists, affect 20% of musicians (Ackermann and Driscoll 2010). Ultrasound reveals increased nerve cross-sectional area (e.g. median nerve >4.8 mm^2 in CTS), while MRI shows nerve oedema.
- *Posture-Related Strain* (Table 7): Sustained postures cause cervical or lumbar strain and spinal deformities like kyphosis, lordosis alterations, or scoliosis (Nyman et al. 2007; Ackermann and Adams 2003). Radiologists use MRI to detect muscle oedema (Fig. 4) and facet hypertrophy, while X-ray reveals abnormal spinal curvatures.
- *Bony/Joint Disorders*: Chronic stress causes osteoarthritis in string players or synovitis in drummers (Zetterberg et al. 1998; Levy et al. 2009). Radiologists use X-ray to detect joint space narrowing and osteophytes, while MRI shows cartilage thinning.
- *Lower Limb Pathologies* (Table 8): Prolonged sitting or kneeling, common in Indian percussionists, causes hip impingement, knee degeneration, or plantar fasciitis (Mishra et al. 2013). Radiologists use MRI arthrography to identify labral tears, X-ray to show knee osteoarthritis, and ultrasound to reveal fascial thickening in plantar fasciitis.
- *Focal Dystonia*: This affects 5%–10% of musicians, often requiring retraining or botulinum toxin (Brandfonbrener 2009). Clinicians

Table 5 Imaging findings for overuse syndromes

Pathology	Imaging modality	Key findings
Rotator cuff tendinopathy	MRI	Tendinosis, partial tears, muscle atrophy
Rotator cuff tendinopathy	Ultrasound	Thickened tendons, hyperaemia
Elbow epicondylitis (Figs. 5 and 6)	MRI	Extensor tendon tears, oedema
Elbow epicondylitis (Fig. 7)	Ultrasound	Hypoechoic tendons, increased vascularity
De Quervain's tenosynovitis	Ultrasound	Fluid, synovial hypertrophy around APL/EPB tendons

Table 6 Imaging findings for nerve compression syndromes

Pathology	Imaging modality	Key findings
Carpal tunnel syndrome	Ultrasound	Increased median nerve cross-sectional area (>4.8 mm^2)
Carpal tunnel syndrome	MRI	Swollen nerve, tenosynovitis
Ulnar neuropathy (Fig. 8)	MRI	Nerve oedema at cubital tunnel
Ulnar neuropathy	Ultrasound	Ulnar nerve subluxation
Thoracic outlet syndrome	MRI neurography	C8–T1 nerve oedema
Thoracic outlet syndrome	Doppler ultrasound	Dynamic arterial compression

Table 7 Imaging findings for spinal deformities

Pathology	Imaging modality	Key findings
Thoracic kyphosis	X-ray	Increased kyphotic angle
Lumbar lordosis/ flattening	MRI	Facet hypertrophy, muscle oedema
Scoliosis	X-ray	Lateral curvature, asymmetric muscle development

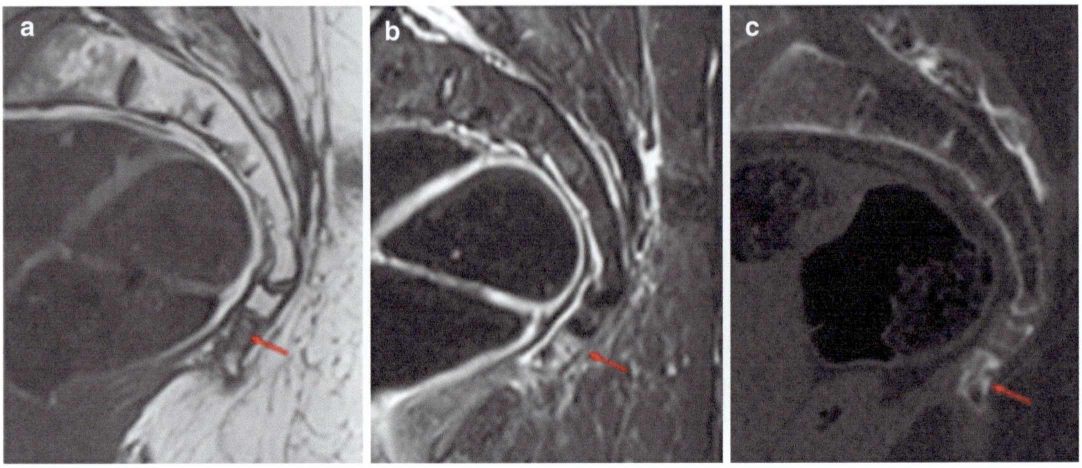

Fig. 4 SagittalT1 (**a**), STIR (**b**), and CT (**c**) showing oedema involving the second coccygeal segment (arrow)

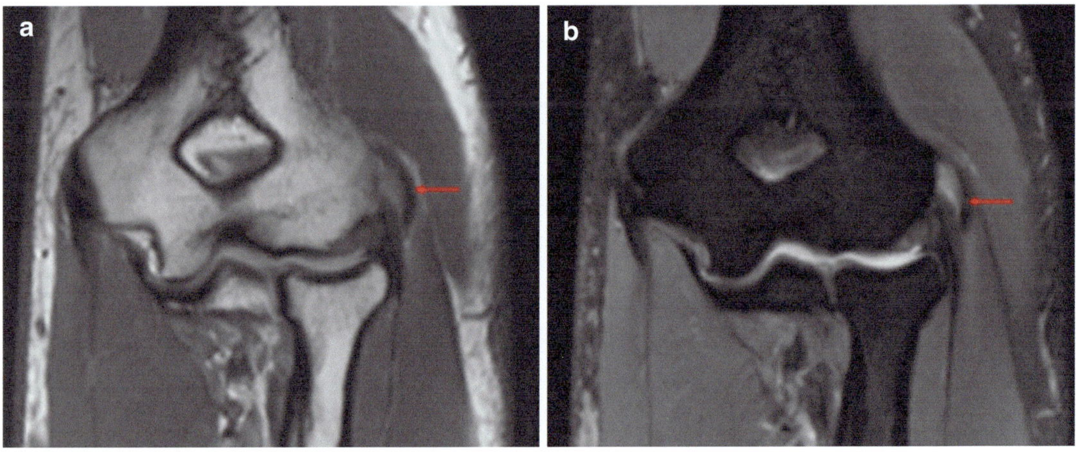

Fig. 5 Coronal PD (**a**) and PDFS (**b**) show oedema and thickening of common extensor origin in keeping with lateral epicondylitis (arrow)

Table 8 Imaging findings for lower limb pathologies

Pathology	Imaging modality	Key findings
Hip impingement/ labral tears	MRI arthrography	Labral fraying, impingement
Knee degeneration	X-ray	Joint space narrowing, osteophytes
Knee degeneration	MRI	Meniscal tears, cartilage thinning
Plantar fasciitis	Ultrasound	Fascial thickening, calcaneal spurs

typically do not use imaging, but functional MRI may provide future insights into neural adaptations.

- *Psychophysiological Factors*: Performance anxiety and stress exacerbate muscle tension, which radiologists observe indirectly through MRI findings of muscle oedema (Kenny and Ackermann 2015).
- *Acute Injuries*: Clinicians manage rare sprains or lacerations with rest, ice, compression, and elevation (RICE) (Levy et al. 2009). They use imaging selectively to rule out fractures or ligament tears.

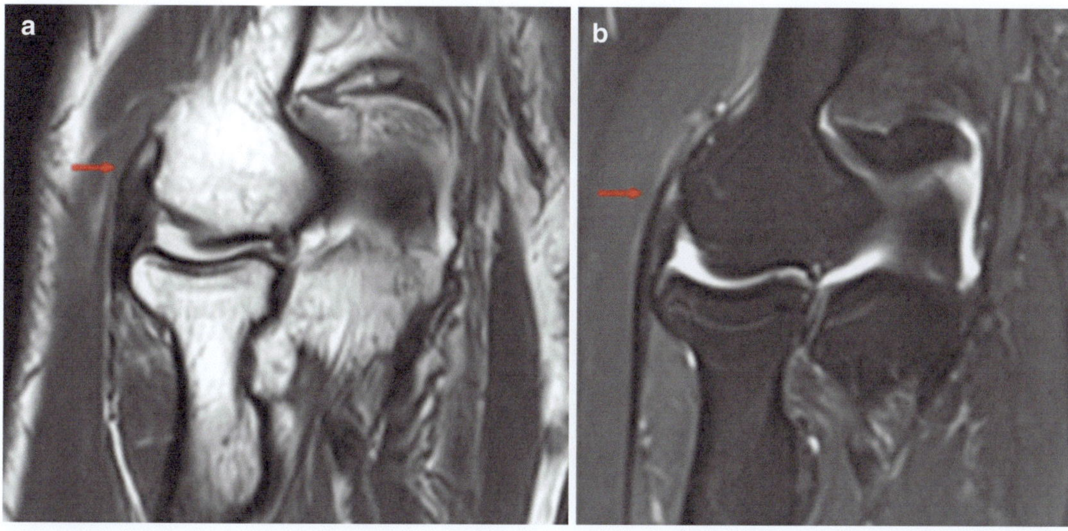

Fig. 6 Coronal PD (**a**) and PDFS (**b**) show oedema and thickening of common extensor origin in keeping with lateral epicondylitis (arrow)

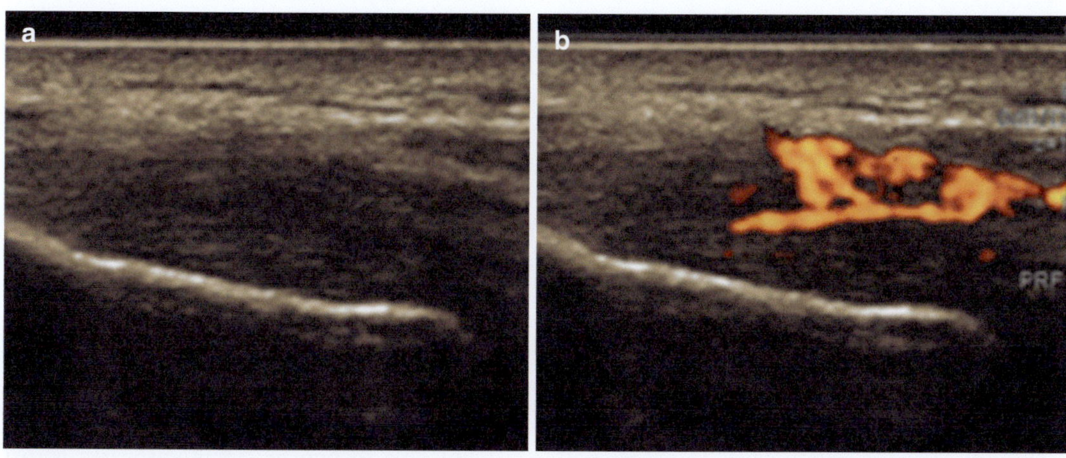

Fig. 7 Longitudinal ultrasound (**a**) and Doppler (**b**) show loss of normal echogenicity with marked increased signal on Doppler of common extensor origin in keeping with lateral epicondylitis

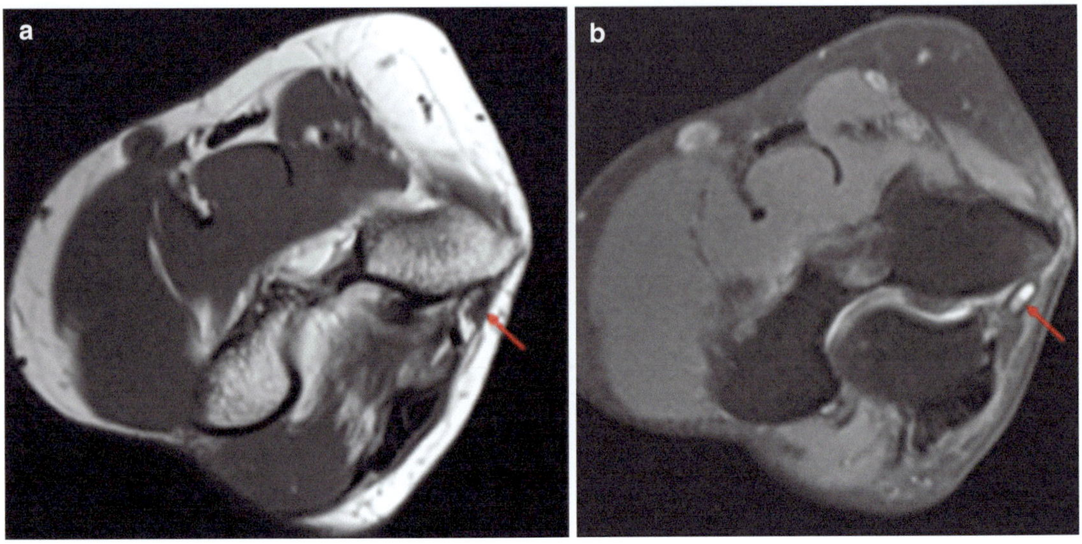

Fig. 8 Axial PD (**a**) and PDFS (**b**) show oedema within the ulnar nerve in the cubital tunnel (arrow)

5 Age-Specific Considerations

PRMDs manifest differently across age groups, influencing how clinicians diagnose and manage them:

- *Paediatric Musicians*: Young musicians, particularly conservatory students, experience a 30%–50% prevalence of pain, with risks to growth plates (Yoshimura et al. 2008). Clinicians use imaging sparingly to minimize radiation exposure but may employ MRI for severe cases to assess soft tissue or joint involvement. Educators prioritize technique training to prevent long-term damage.
- *Adult Musicians*: Adults face the highest PRMD prevalence due to intense practice schedules, with tendinopathies and nerve entrapments being common (Zaza and Farewell 1997). Radiologists use MRI and ultrasound to confirm diagnoses, such as rotator cuff tendinopathy or CTS, guiding targeted interventions.
- *Older Musicians*: Degenerative changes, such as osteoarthritis or disc degeneration, complicate PRMDs in older musicians (Zetterberg et al. 1998). Radiologists use X-rays to detect bony changes and MRI to identify cartilage loss or disc pathology, informing adapted techniques to prolong careers.

Clinicians recognize symptoms early across all age groups to prevent chronicity, with imaging playing a key role in confirming diagnoses and guiding treatment (Barton et al. 2008).

Other Injuries Seen in Musicians: (All Images Source: Author) (Figs. 9, 10, 11, 12, 13, 14, 15, and 16)

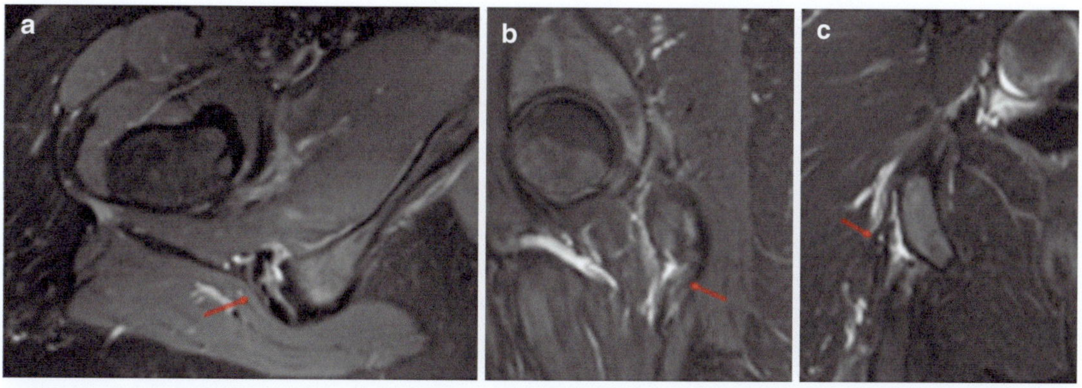

Fig. 9 PDFS axial (**a**), sagittal (**b**), and coronal (**c**) showing tendinopathy of right hamstring at its ischial origin with mild ischial bursitis (arrow)

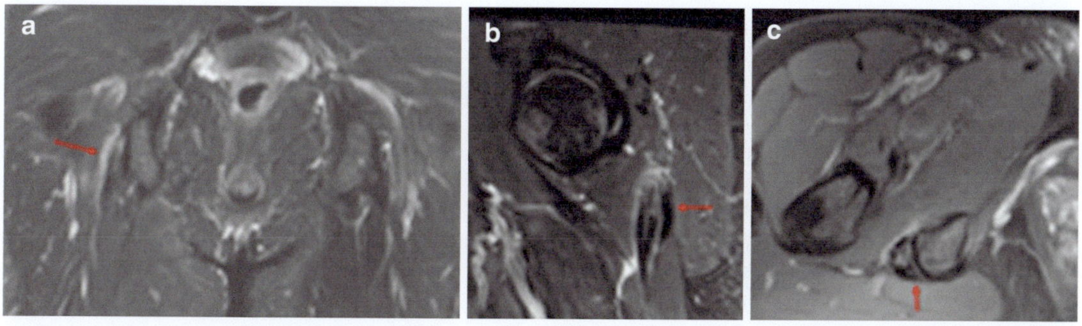

Fig. 10 PDFS coronal (**a**), sagittal (**b**), and axial (**c**) showing tendinopathy of right hamstrings at its ischial origin (arrow)

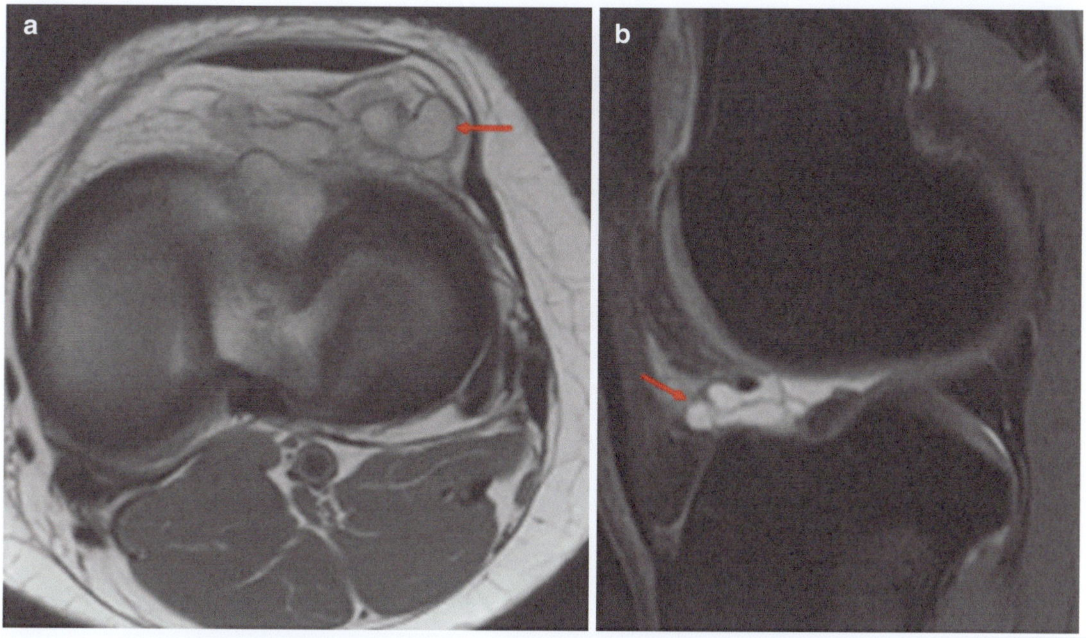

Fig. 11 Axial PD (**a**) and sagittal PDFS (**b**) demonstrating Hoffa's fat pad ganglion (arrow)

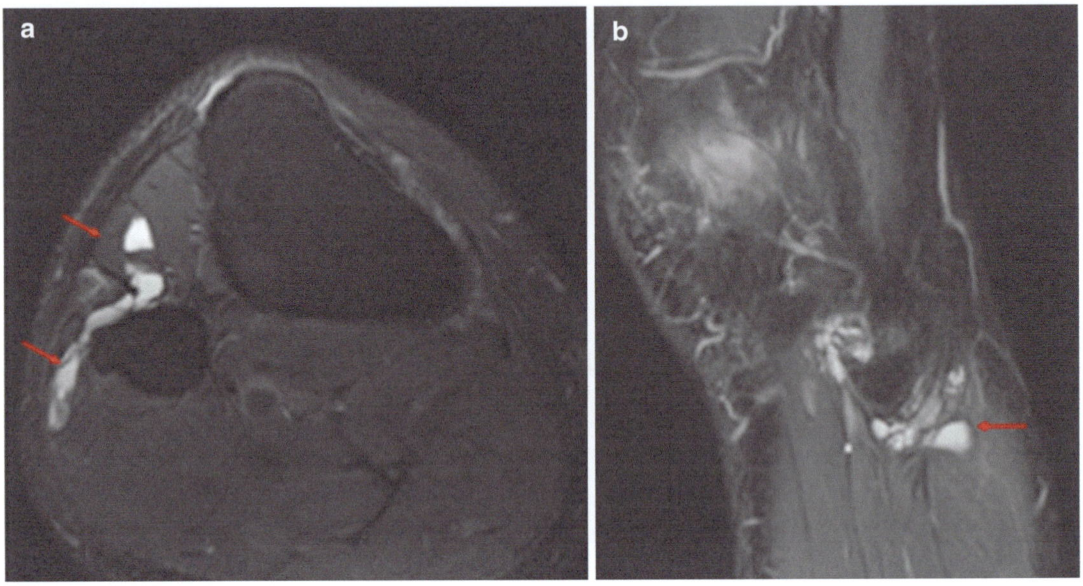

Fig. 12 Axial PDFS (**a**) and sagittal PDFS (**b**) show intraneural ganglion of common peroneal nerve (arrow)

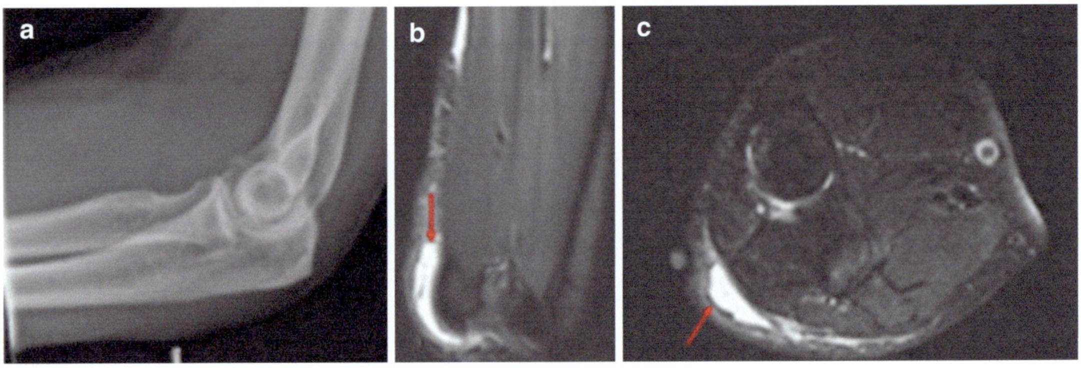

Fig. 13 Lateral radiograph of elbow (**a**) shows soft tissue swelling in relation to olecranon. Sagittal PDFS (**b**) and axial PDFS (**c**) show olecranon bursitis (arrow)

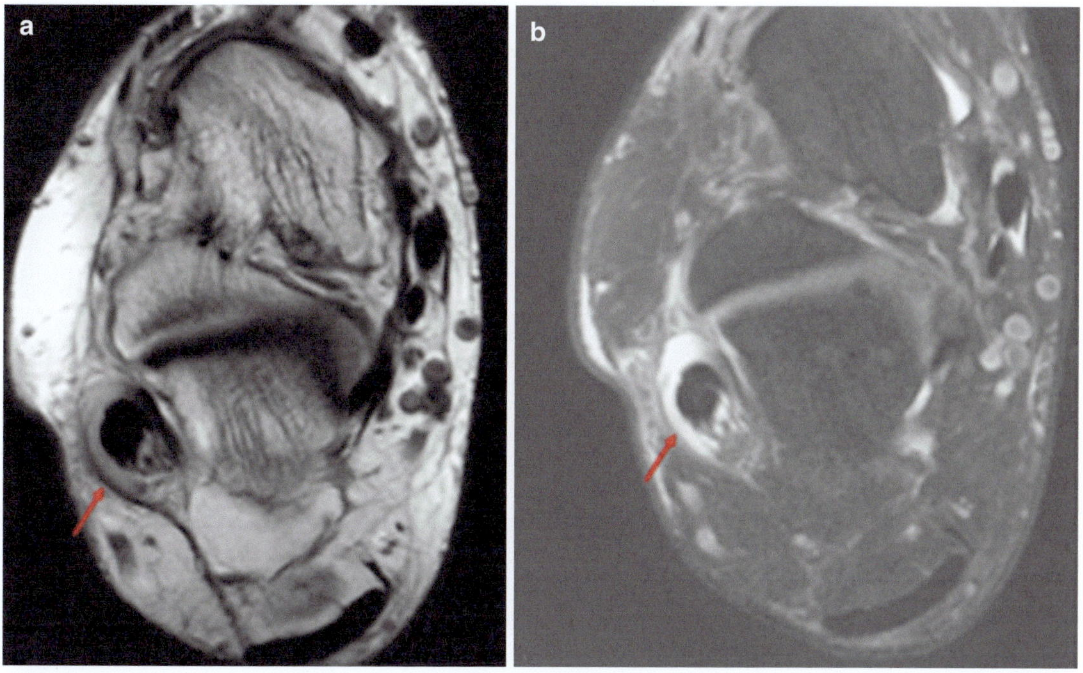

Fig. 14 Axial PD (**a**) and PDFS (**b**) show peroneal tenosynovitis (arrow)

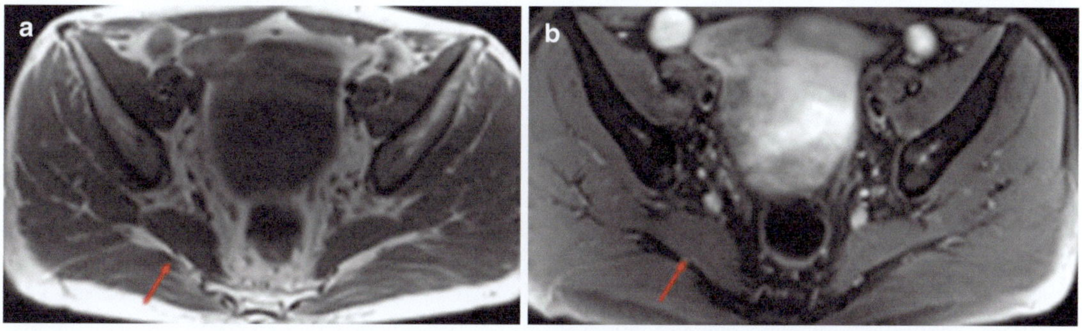

Fig. 15 Axial PD (**a**) and PDFS (**b**) show bulkier right piriformis muscle in keeping with piriformis syndrome (arrow)

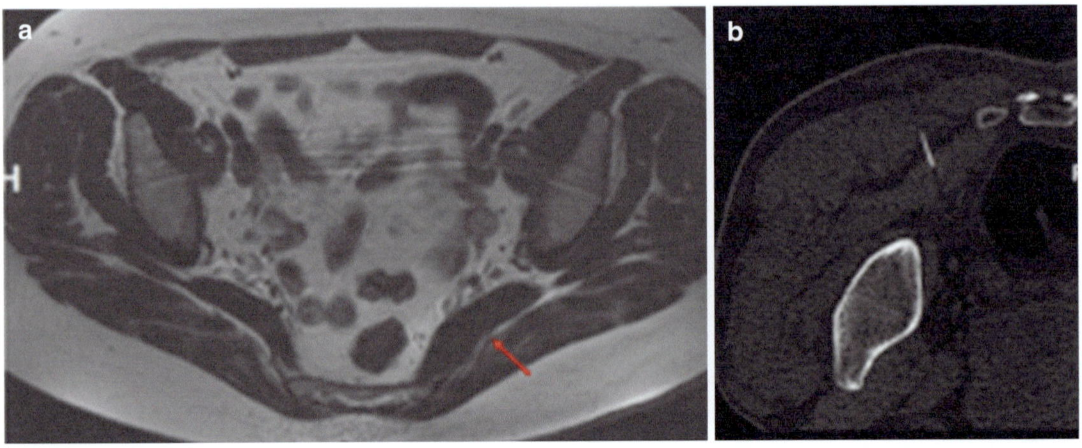

Fig. 16 Axial PD (**a**) shows bulkier left piriformis muscle in keeping with piriformis syndrome (arrow). This was treated with CT-guided injection (**b**)

6 Diagnostic Approach

Clinicians diagnose PRMDs through a multifaceted approach, integrating a detailed, instrument-specific history, comprehensive physical examination, and targeted imaging or electrodiagnostics. This method addresses each instrument's unique biomechanical stressors and accurately identifies underlying pathologies.

- *History*: Clinicians gather details on practice duration, symptom onset, and psychosocial factors, such as performance anxiety, which may worsen symptoms (Hoppmann and Patrone 1989; Kenny and Ackermann 2015). Night pain or paraesthesias suggest nerve entrapment, such as carpal tunnel syndrome (CTS) or cubital tunnel syndrome (Brandfonbrener 2009).
- *Physical Examination*: Clinicians perform thorough assessments of posture, range of motion, muscle strength, and tenderness. They mimic the musician's playing position to identify biomechanical faults, such as shoulder elevation in violinists or wrist deviation in pianists (Ackermann and Adams 2003). Provocation tests, like Phalen's for CTS or Tinel's for ulnar neuropathy, confirm nerve entrapment (Kaufman-Cohen and Ratzon 2011).
- *Imaging and Electrodiagnostics*:
  - *X-ray*: Detects bony abnormalities, such as osteophytes, joint space narrowing, or spinal deformities like scoliosis or kyphosis.
  - *MRI*: Serves as the gold standard for soft tissue evaluation, revealing muscle oedema, tendon tears, disc bulges, or nerve compression.
  - *Ultrasound*: Provides dynamic assessment of tendons (e.g. hyperaemia in tendinopathy) and nerves (e.g. median nerve enlargement in CTS). Doppler ultrasound evaluates vascular compression in thoracic outlet syndrome.
  - *CT*: Assesses bony structures, such as TMJ osteophytes or calcaneal spurs in plantar fasciitis.
  - *Electromyography (EMG)*: Confirms neuropathy in severe cases, particularly for nerve entrapment syndromes (Ackermann and Driscoll 2010).
  - *MRI Neurography*: Visualizes nerve oedema in conditions like thoracic outlet syndrome.
- *Specialized Testing*: Clinicians use motion capture systems for real-time biomechanical analysis and validated questionnaires, such as the Musicians' Health and Wellness Survey, to track symptom progression (Ackermann and Driscoll 2010; Steinmetz et al. 2020).

7 Non-surgical Management

Clinicians prioritize conservative management for PRMDs, tailoring interventions to specific pathologies and instruments based on imaging findings. They employ the following strategies, often in combination, to relieve symptoms and restore function:

- *Activity Modification and Practice Adjustments*: Clinicians recommend reducing practice duration, incorporating regular breaks, and avoiding extreme joint positions to minimize biomechanical stress (Zaza and Farewell 1997; Bragge et al. 2006). For example, violinists with trapezius myalgia benefit from shorter practice sessions, guided by MRI findings of muscle oedema to determine rest requirements.
- *Physiotherapy and Strengthening Protocols*: Physiotherapists stretch tight muscles (e.g. trapezius in violinists) and strengthen weak areas (e.g. rotator cuff in string players) (Ackermann and Adams 2003). Ultrasound monitors tendon recovery, while targeted exercises, such as scapular stabilization for shoulder impingement, improve outcomes (Steinmetz et al. 2015).
- *Ergonomic Retraining and Equipment Use*: Clinicians prescribe adjustable chairs, shoulder rests for violinists, or the Alexander Technique to reduce muscle tension and improve posture (Ackermann and Adams 2003; Rickert et al. 2013). For Indian musicians, cushions or modified seating alleviate hip and lumbar stress from cross-legged postures.
- *Pharmacologic and Modality-Based Interventions*: Clinicians administer non-steroidal anti-inflammatory drugs (NSAIDs) to manage acute inflammation and cautiously use corticosteroid injections for severe tendinopathies, ensuring MRI confirms no significant structural damage (Brandfonbrener 2009). Limited evidence supports acupuncture as an adjunct (Steinmetz et al. 2015).
- *Psychosocial Support and Return-to-Play Protocols*: Psychologists provide cognitive-behavioural therapy (CBT) to address performance anxiety, which exacerbates muscle tension observable on MRI (Kenny and Ackermann 2015). Clinicians guide gradual resumption of practice with pain monitoring to ensure safe return to performance (Zaza and Farewell 1997).

The "Sound Practice" initiative integrates education, biomechanical feedback, and multidisciplinary care, significantly reducing PRMD incidence (Rickert et al. 2014).

8 Surgical Interventions

Surgeons reserve surgical intervention for severe or refractory PRMD cases where conservative management fails (Hoppmann and Patrone 1989). They perform the following procedures:

- *Nerve Decompression*: Surgeons conduct carpal tunnel release for pianists with CTS or cubital tunnel release for flutists with ulnar neuropathy. Preoperative MRI identifies the extent of nerve compression, while postoperative ultrasound monitors recovery.
- *Tendon/Joint Surgery*: Surgeons perform De Quervain's release for keyboardists or rotator cuff repair for string players. MRI guides surgical planning by delineating tendon tears or joint pathology.
- *Ligament Repairs*: Surgeons address rare traumatic injuries, using X-rays to ensure proper alignment post-surgery.

Red Flags for Surgical Referral

- Persistent night pain unrelieved by rest.
- Progressive muscle weakness or atrophy.
- EMG-confirmed severe nerve entrapment.
- Failure of 8–12 weeks of conservative management.

Postoperative rehabilitation emphasizes early motion to prevent stiffness, with full recovery typically taking 3–6 months. Surgeons use postoperative X-rays or ultrasound to confirm proper healing and alignment (Steinmetz et al. 2015).

9 Case Examples

To illustrate the integration of orthopaedic and radiological approaches, the following case examples highlight common PRMDs, their imaging findings, and management strategies:

1. *Case 1: Violinist with Neck Pain*
   A 25-year-old professional violinist presents with right-sided neck and shoulder pain after prolonged rehearsals. Clinicians identify trapezius strain and limited cervical range of motion during physical examination. Radiologists use MRI to confirm muscle oedema in the cervical region, consistent with strain (Nyman et al. 2007). Clinicians prescribe rest, the Alexander Technique to improve posture, and scapular stabilization exercises. Symptoms resolve within 6 weeks, with follow-up ultrasound confirming reduced muscle inflammation (Ackermann and Adams 2003).
2. *Case 2: Pianist with Wrist Pain*
   A 30-year-old pianist reports numbness and tingling in the right hand, worsened by playing. Radiologists use ultrasound to reveal an enlarged median nerve (>4.8 mm^2), confirming CTS (Bragge et al. 2006). After failed conservative management with splinting and physiotherapy, surgeons perform carpal tunnel release. Postoperative MRI confirms nerve decompression, and rehabilitation restores function within 4 months (Steinmetz et al. 2015).
3. *Case 3: Tabla Player with Back Pain*
   A 45-year-old tabla player presents with chronic low back pain from cross-legged sitting. Radiologists use MRI to reveal a lumbar disc bulge with Modic changes, indicating degeneration (Chandran et al. 2022). Clinicians prescribe core strengthening exercises, posture adjustments with cushioned seating, and NSAIDs. Symptoms resolve in 2 months, with follow-up X-ray showing stable spondylotic changes (Mishra et al. 2013).
4. *Case 4: Flutist with Elbow Paraesthesias*
   A 38-year-old flutist reports elbow paraesthesias and weakness. Radiologists use MRI to confirm ulnar nerve oedema at the cubital tunnel, diagnosing cubital tunnel syndrome (Kaufman-Cohen and Ratzon 2011). Clinicians prescribe conservative management with an elbow sleeve, nerve gliding exercises, and activity modification, improving symptoms within 3 months. Ultrasound verifies reduced nerve swelling (Steinmetz et al. 2015).

10 Preventive Strategies and Multidisciplinary Management

Clinicians and educators adopt a proactive, multidisciplinary approach to prevent PRMDs, addressing biomechanical, ergonomic, and psychosocial factors. They implement the following evidence-based strategies:

- *Education*: Educators teach musicians proper posture, technique, and the importance of regular rest breaks to minimize biomechanical stress (Zaza and Farewell 1997). Workshops on injury prevention, especially for students, reduce PRMD incidence.
- *Ergonomic Adjustments*: Clinicians recommend instrument-specific equipment, such as adjustable chairs, shoulder rests for violinists, or padded mats for percussionists, to reduce strain (Ackermann and Adams 2003). For Indian musicians, modified seating arrangements alleviate hip and lumbar stress from cross-legged postures.
- *Physical Conditioning*: Musicians engage in regular exercise, including yoga or Pilates, to enhance flexibility, strength, and endurance, reducing overuse injury risks (Barton et al. 2008). Core strengthening benefits percussionists and keyboardists particularly.
- *Multidisciplinary Screening*: Clinicians conduct routine screenings, incorporating physical examinations and selective imaging (e.g. ultrasound for tendon thickening), to detect subclinical PRMDs and enable early intervention (Steinmetz et al. 2020).
- *Policy Measures*: Institutions and orchestras implement policies to limit excessive practice schedules and promote rest, reducing cumulative stress (Rickert et al. 2013).

Box 1: Preventive Strategies for PRMDs

- Educate musicians on posture, technique, and rest breaks.
- Use ergonomic equipment tailored to specific instruments.
- Promote physical conditioning through yoga or Pilates.
- Conduct multidisciplinary screenings to detect early PRMDs.
- Implement policies to avoid excessive practice schedules. *Caption*: Evidence-based strategies to prevent PRMDs, supporting sustainable musical careers.

11 Future Directions

Researchers and clinicians advance PRMD management through emerging technologies and studies. Wearable sensors, such as Upright Go, provide real-time feedback on spinal posture, reducing flexion in pianists and other musicians (Steinmetz et al. 2020). Motion-capture systems analyse biomechanics in detail, identifying subtle technique faults that contribute to injury. Functional MRI offers potential insights into neural adaptations in musicians with chronic pain or focal dystonia, guiding novel interventions.

Researchers need prospective studies to validate these technologies, particularly for Indian classical instruments with unique biomechanical demands (Chandran et al. 2022). Randomized controlled trials on rehabilitation protocols, such as physiotherapy or ergonomic interventions, would strengthen the evidence base. Educators should develop injury prevention curricula for music schools and orchestras to reduce PRMD incidence, ensuring musicians' long-term health (Rickert et al. 2014; Sanderson et al. 2007).

12 Conclusion

Performance-related musculoskeletal disorders challenge instrumental musicians due to the repetitive, forceful, and often asymmetric demands of their instruments. Clinicians integrate orthopaedic principles—biomechanical analysis, clinical diagnosis, and rehabilitation—with radiological insights from MRI, ultrasound, X-ray, and CT to achieve precise diagnoses and tailor interventions to each musician's needs. This chapter provides a comprehensive framework for understanding PRMDs, from their epidemiology and biomechanical origins to their diagnosis, management, and prevention. It emphasizes the unique challenges Indian classical musicians face due to traditional postures that heighten spinal and lower limb pathology risks.

Radiologists use imaging to visualize biomechanical stress consequences, from muscle oedema and tendon tears to nerve compression and joint degeneration. Clinicians prioritize conservative management, including physiotherapy, ergonomic retraining, and activity modification, reserving surgical interventions for severe cases. Educators and clinicians implement preventive strategies, supported by education, ergonomic adjustments, and technologies like wearable sensors, to ensure sustainable musical careers.

This integrated orthopaedic and radiological approach equips healthcare professionals to support musicians effectively, bridging clinical assessment and advanced imaging. By addressing PRMDs holistically, clinicians help musicians maintain their artistry without sacrificing physical health, fostering longevity in a demanding yet rewarding profession.

References

Ackermann B, Adams R (2003) Physical characteristics and pain patterns of skilled violinists. Med Probl Perform Art 18:65–71

Ackermann B, Driscoll T (2010) Development of a new instrument for musicians' health: the Musicians' Health and Wellness Survey. Med Probl Perform Art 25(4):147–155. https://doi.org/10.21091/mppa.2010.4028

Baadjou VA et al (2016) Health problems in musicians—a systematic review on prevalence and associated risk factors. Musculoskelet Sci Pract 27:18–29. https://doi.org/10.1016/j.math.2016.03.004

Barton R et al (2008) Occupational performance issues and predictors of dysfunction in college instrumentalists. Med Probl Perform Art 23:72–78

Bragge P, Bialocerkowski A, McMeeken J (2006) A systematic review of prevalence and risk factors associated with playing-related musculoskeletal disorders in pianists. Occup Med (Lond) 56:28–38. https://doi.org/10.1093/occmed/kqi177

Brandfonbrener AG (2009) Musculoskeletal problems of instrumental musicians. Hand Clin 25(1):101–112. https://doi.org/10.1016/j.hcl.2008.09.006

Chandran A et al (2022) Musculoskeletal disorders in Indian percussionists: an observational study. Indian J Occup Environ Med 26(2):81–90

Davies J, Mangion S (2002) Predictors of pain and other musculoskeletal symptoms among professional instrumental musicians: elucidating specific effects. Med Probl Perform Art 17:155–168

Fotiadis D, Fotiadou EG, Kokaridas DG, Mylonas AC (2013) Prevalence of musculoskeletal disorders in professional symphony orchestra musicians in Greece. Med Probl Perform Art 28:91–95

Hoppmann RA, Patrone NA (1989) A review of musculoskeletal problems in instrumental musicians. Semin Arthritis Rheum 19(2):117–126. https://doi.org/10.1016/0049-0172(89)90035-0

Kaufman-Cohen Y, Ratzon NZ (2011) Correlation between risk factors and musculoskeletal disorders among classical musicians. Occup Med (Lond) 61(2):90–95. https://doi.org/10.1093/occmed/kqq196

Kenny D, Ackermann B (2015) Performance-related musculoskeletal pain, depression and music performance anxiety in professional orchestral musicians: a population study. Psychol Music 43:43–60. https://doi.org/10.1177/0305735613493953

Leaver R, Harris EC, Palmer KT (2011) Musculoskeletal pain in elite professional musicians from British symphony orchestras. Occup Med (Lond) 61:549–555. https://doi.org/10.1093/occmed/kqr129

Levy JJ, Lounsbury JW, Kent KN (2009) Big five personality traits and marching music injuries. Med Probl Perform Art 24:135–140

Mishra W et al (2013) Playing-related musculoskeletal disorders among Indian tabla players. Med Probl Perform Art 28(2):107–111. https://doi.org/10.21091/mppa.2013.2019

Nyman T et al (2007) Work postures and neck-shoulder pain among orchestra musicians. Am J Ind Med 50:370–376. https://doi.org/10.1002/ajim.20454

Paarup HM et al (2011) Prevalence and consequences of musculoskeletal symptoms in symphony orchestra musicians vary by gender: a cross-sectional study. BMC Musculoskelet Disord 12:223. https://doi.org/10.1186/1471-2474-12-223

Rickert DL, Barrett MS, Ackermann BJ (2013) Injury and the orchestral environment: part I. The role of work organisation and psychosocial factors in injury risk. Med Probl Perform Art 28:219–229

Rickert DL, Barrett MS, Ackermann BJ (2014) Injury and the orchestral environment: part II. Organisational culture, behavioural norms, and attitudes to injury. Med Probl Perform Art 29(3):133–140. https://doi.org/10.21091/mppa.2014.3027

Roach KE, Martinez MA, Anderson N (1994) Musculoskeletal pain in student instrumentalists: a comparison with the general student population. Med Probl Perform Art 9:125–130

Sanderson S, Tatt ID, Higgins JP (2007) Tools for assessing quality and susceptibility to bias in observational studies in epidemiology: a systematic review and annotated bibliography. Int J Epidemiol 36:666–676. https://doi.org/10.1093/ije/dym018

Silva AG, La FMB, Afreixo V (2015) Pain prevalence in instrumental musicians: a systematic review. Med Probl Perform Art 30:8–19

Steinmetz A et al (2015) Frequency, severity and predictors of playing-related musculoskeletal pain in professional orchestral musicians in Germany. Clin Rheumatol 34:965–973. https://doi.org/10.1007/s10067-013-2465-5

Steinmetz A et al (2020) Symptoms and risk factors of musculoskeletal disorders in professional musicians: a prospective study. J Occup Med Toxicol 15:Article 9. https://doi.org/10.1186/s12995-020-00266-8

Yoshimura E et al (2008) Risk factors for musculoskeletal disorders in university student instrumental musicians: a cross-sectional study. BMC Musculoskelet Disord 9:116. https://doi.org/10.1186/1471-2474-9-116

Zaza C (1998) Playing-related musculoskeletal disorders in musicians: a systematic review of incidence and prevalence. Can Med Assoc J 158(8):1019–1025

Zaza C, Farewell VT (1997) Musicians' playing-related musculoskeletal disorders: an examination of risk factors. Am J Ind Med 32:292–300

Zaza C, Charles C, Muszynski A (1998) The meaning of playing-related musculoskeletal disorders to classical musicians. Soc Sci Med 47:2013–2023

Zetterberg C, Backlund H, Karlsson J, Werner H. Olsson, L (1998) Musculoskeletal problems among male and female music students. Medical Problems of Performing Artists 13(4):160–166. http://www.jstor.org/stable/45440347

Foot and Ankle Non-traumatic Disorders: Indian Classical Musicians to Take Note

P. R. Krishna Prasad, Akanksh Chokkapu, Siva Sai Gorle, and Durgananda Lahari Bhamidipaty

Contents

P. R. K. Prasad
Department of Orthopaedics, KMC, Manipal, India

A. Chokkapu · S. S. Gorle
Department of Radiodiagnosis, NRIIMS, Visakhapatnam, India

D. L. Bhamidipaty (✉)
Department of Industrial Biotechnology, Manipal Institute of Technology, Manipal, India

Med Radiol Diagn Imaging (2025)
https://doi.org/10.1007/174_2025_657,
Published Online: 29 November 2025

Abstract

Indian classical musicians often spend prolonged hours in static and repetitive postures, particularly in cross-legged sitting positions during practice and performance. Such long-term occupational demands predispose them to a variety of musculoskeletal problems involving the lower limbs, especially the foot and ankle, which serve as the final point of weight transmission and balance. Non-traumatic disorders in this region may present as chronic pain, deformities, enthesopathies, nerve compressions, and vascular compromise. These conditions are often under-recognized, as the artistic demands and cultural context of performance tend to overshadow the physical strain on the musician's body. Early identification and management are crucial in preventing long-term disability and ensuring career longevity. This chapter highlights the common foot and ankle disorders seen in Indian classical musicians, their biomechanical basis, clinical features, radiological correlates, and possible preventive and rehabilitative strategies. By raising awareness among performers, teachers, and healthcare professionals, this work aims to integrate ergonomics and musculoskeletal health into the training and practice of Indian classical music.

1 Introduction

Prolonged hours of practice and performance are integral to Indian classical musicians. The cross-legged sitting for hours continuously in these postures for periods as long as a few decades makes these individuals prone to many disorders of the lower limb (Table 1). However, the ankle and foot, which are at the fag end of weight transmission of the body, are more vulnerable. These performers often perform barefoot, as a token of respect whether towards elders, gurus, or in temple premises. This makes them prone to pain and disability, which, if neglected, can lead to deformity.

In this chapter, we are going to touch upon various non-traumatic disorders which can affect the foot and ankle. In Indian classical musicians, these disorders can interfere with day-to-day activities as well as their performing arts.

Table 1 Postural and dynamic risk factors for ankle injury
Biomechanical stressors and injury risks by instrument in Indian classical musicians

Instrument	Playing posture	Static ankle stress	Role of talam	Dynamic ankle stress	Injury risk profile
Tabla/Mridangam	Cross-legged	Plantarflexion/inversion; CPN compression	–	–	High CPN palsy risk; moderate soft tissue strain.
Carnatic Violin/Flute	Cross-legged	Plantarflexion/inversion; CPN compression	Repetitive foot tapping	Dorsi/plantarflexion; impact loading	High risk for CPN palsy, tendinopathies TTS, stress fractures.
Sitar/Sarod	Cross-legged (one leg raised)	Asymmetric loading; plantarflexion/inversion	–	–	Moderate CPN palsy, postural strain risk.
Harmonium	Cross-legged	Plantarflexion/inversion; CPN compression	–	–	High CPN palsy risk; moderate soft tissue strain.

Source: Author

2 Common Peroneal Nerve (CPN) Palsy (Tables 2 and 3)

2.1 Anatomy and Pathophysiology

The CPN, a sciatic nerve branch, lies exposed at the fibular head. Cross-legged sitting for over 120 min compresses the nerve, causing venous obstruction, edema, and ischemia, leading to neuropraxia (Chandra et al. 2017; Yu et al. 2013).

2.2 Clinical Presentation

CPN palsy causes foot drop, with weak ankle dorsiflexion and eversion, and numbness or tingling over the foot dorsum and lateral shin. Pain is often minimal (Yu et al. 2013).

2.3 Diagnosis and Differential

Clinicians diagnose CPN palsy via history of cross-legged sitting and a positive Tinel's sign at

Table 2 Differential diagnosis of ankle neuropathies

Feature	CPN Palsy	TTS	L5 Radiculopathy
Nerve	Common Peroneal	Posterior tibial	L5 Spinal Root
Mechanism	Compression at fibular head	Tarsal tunnel compression	Nerve root compression
Sensory Symptoms	Foot dorsum, lateral shin	Plantar foot, toes	Lateral leg, foot dorsum
Motor Deficits	Foot drop	Intrinsic foot weakness (late)	Foot drop, inversion/abduction weakness
Reflexes	Normal	Normal	Diminished (e.g., medial hamstring)
Key Sign	Tinel's at fibular head	Tinel's at medial ankle	Straight leg raise, back pain

Source: Author

Table 3 Imaging findings in ankle injuries
Radiological features of ankle injuries in Indian classical musicians, with key findings emphasized

Condition	Radiography	Ultrasound	MRI	CT
CPN Palsy	Normal	Nerve flattening at fibular head	Nerve edema, compression	
TTS	Normal	Tibial nerve compression, tenosynovitis	Nerve edema, cysts	
Tendinopathies	Normal	Thickened, hypoechoic tendon; anisotropy pitfall	T2 hyperintensity, thickening	–
Stress Fractures	Negative early; later periosteal reaction	–	Periosteal/bone marrow edema, fracture line	Complex fractures, pre-surgical planning
Lateral Malleolar Bursitis	Normal	Fluid-filled bursa, thickened walls	Bursal inflammation, abscess	–
Achilles Tendinopathy	Haglund deformity, intratendinous osteophytes	Tendinosis, calcific foci	Tendon thickening, calcific deposits	–

Source: Author

the fibular head. Electrodiagnostic studies confirm lesion location (Chandra et al. 2017). L5 radiculopathy is ruled out by weak ankle inversion, hip abduction, and back pain/sciatica.

Radiology Spotlight:

- Ultrasound: Detects CPN flattening at the fibular head, especially during dynamic cross-legged posture assessment.
- MRI: Shows nerve edema or compression, useful in atypical cases.
- Pitfall: Normal imaging does not rule out early neuropraxia; correlate with electrodiagnostics.

Key Teaching Points:

- Ask about cross-legged sitting in musicians with foot drop to rule out CPN palsy.
- A positive Tinel's sign at the fibular head is diagnostic.
- Ultrasound confirms dynamic CPN compression.
- Electrodiagnostics distinguish peripheral from spinal etiologies.

3 Tarsal Tunnel Syndrome (TTS) (Tables 2 and 3)

3.1 Anatomy and Pathophysiology

The posterior tibial nerve, within the tarsal tunnel, is compressed by talam-induced tenosynovitis or pronation. Trauma contributes in 43% of cases (Ahmad et al. 2017).

3.2 Clinical Presentation

TTS presents with burning or tingling plantar foot pain, worsening with talam and at night. Late cases show intrinsic foot muscle weakness (Quirk 2008).

3.3 Diagnosis and Differential

A positive Tinel's sign at the medial ankle and tenderness confirm TTS (Fig. 1). Plantar fasciitis lacks neuropathic symptoms. Imaging identifies compressive lesions (Ahmad et al. 2017; Quirk 2008).

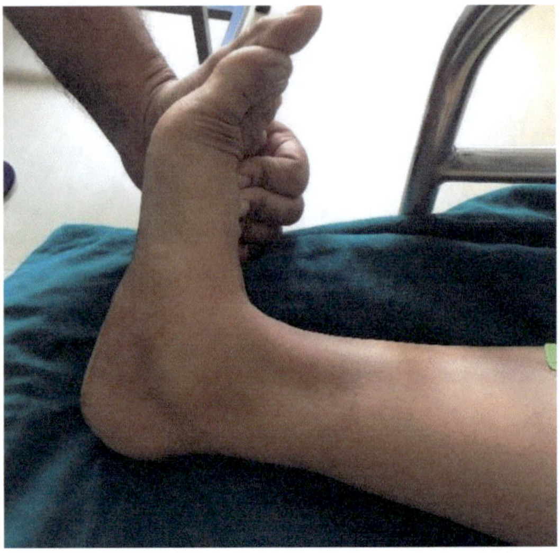

Fig. 1 Stress test for confirmation of TTS. (Source: Author)

Radiology Spotlight:

- MRI: Detects nerve edema or compressive cysts in the tarsal tunnel (Fig. 2).
- Ultrasound: Shows tibial nerve compression or tenosynovitis.
- Pitfall: Normal electrodiagnostics may occur; imaging is critical for confirmation.

Key Teaching Points:

- Suspect TTS in musicians with plantar foot pain during talam.
- Neuropathic pain distinguishes TTS from plantar fasciitis.
- MRI or ultrasound detects compressive causes like cysts.
- Early diagnosis prevents muscle weakness.

Treatment:

- Surgical decompression of tarsal tunnel in cases of compressive lesions like cysts (Fig. 3).
- Physiotherapy and medical management to alleviate pain.

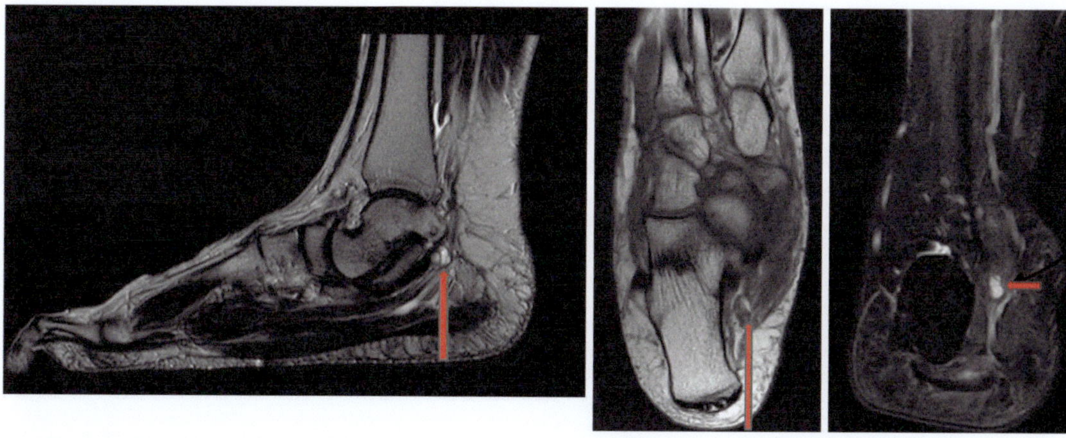

Fig. 2 MRI Ankle (Sagittal, Axial & Coronal) shows small ganglion cyst ~1 × 0.7 cms noted in the tarsal tunnel, between posterior tibial nerve and artery abutting the nerve along its medial aspect. (Source: Author)

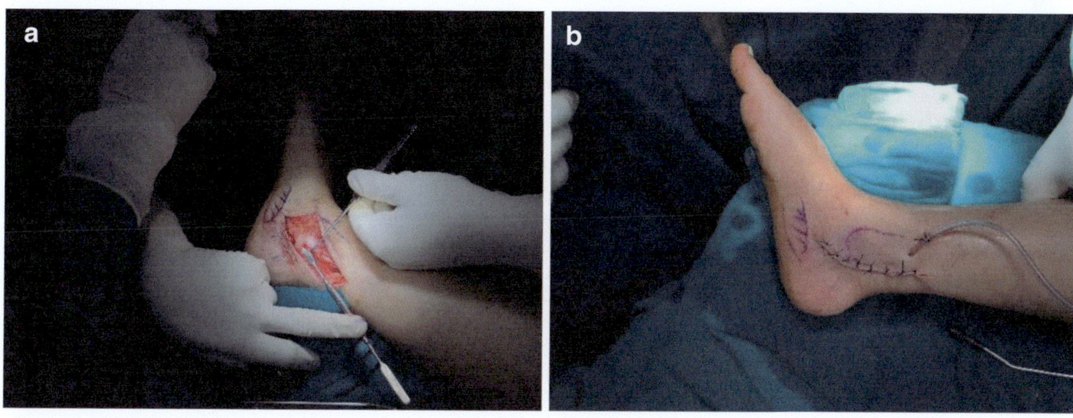

Fig. 3 (**a**) Surgical release of tarsal tunnel, (**b**) Post decompression. (Source: Author)

4 Posterior Tibialis Tendinopathy (Table 3)

4.1 Anatomy and Function

The posterior tibialis tendon (PTTD, defined as posterior tibialis tendinopathy) supports the medial arch, plantarflexes, and inverts the foot (Quirk 2008).

4.2 Pathophysiology

Talam's repetitive plantarflexion induces microtrauma in the hypovascular zone behind the medial malleolus, progressing to tendinosis. Risk factors include pes planus and female sex (aged 40–50) (Quirk 2008; Simpson and Howard 2009).

4.3 Clinical Presentation

Posterior tibialis tendinopathy causes medial ankle and foot pain with swelling, worsening with activity. Progressive cases show flatfoot deformity and a positive "too many toes" sign. The single-leg heel raise test confirms weakness (Quirk 2008).

Radiology Spotlight:

- MRI: Shows T2 hyperintensity and tendon thickening, indicating tendinosis.
- Ultrasound: Detects hypoechoic tendon thickening.
- Pitfall: Anisotropy may mimic pathology; adjust probe angle.

Key Teaching Points:

- Posterior tibialis tendinopathy mimics TTS but lacks neuropathic symptoms.
- The single-leg heel raise test is diagnostic.
- MRI confirms tendon thickening and hyperintensity.
- Early intervention prevents flatfoot deformity.

5 Anterior Tibialis Tendinopathy (Table 3)

5.1 Anatomy and Function

The anterior tibialis tendon enables dorsiflexion and inversion (Quirk 2008).

5.2 Pathophysiology

Repetitive dorsiflexion during talam causes microtrauma, leading to inflammation, similar to hill-running injuries (Quirk 2008; Simpson and Howard 2009).

5.3 Clinical Presentation

Anteromedial ankle pain, tenderness, and swelling worsen with dorsiflexion. Crepitus may occur (Quirk 2008).

Radiology Spotlight:

- Ultrasound: Detects hypoechoic tendon thickening at the insertion.
- MRI: Shows tendon edema or thickening.
- Pitfall: Anisotropy requires careful probe adjustment.

Key Teaching Points:

- Link anterior tibialis tendinopathy to talam-induced dorsiflexion.
- Pain with resisted dorsiflexion confirms diagnosis.
- Ultrasound detects tendon thickening.
- Eccentric exercises promote healing.

6 Bone Stress Injuries (Table 3)

6.1 Pathophysiology

Talam impacts cause bone resorption, leading to microfractures if repair lags. Muscle fatigue increases skeletal stress. Athletic studies support an inferred risk, though musician-specific data are lacking (Warden et al. 2014).

6.2 Common Locations

Likely sites include metatarsals (2–3), calcaneus, navicular, and tibia. High-risk fractures (e.g., navicular) may need surgery (Warden et al. 2014).

6.3 Clinical Presentation

Activity-dependent bone pain with pinpoint tenderness is diagnostic. Early radiographs may be negative, requiring MRI (Warden et al. 2014).

Radiology Spotlight:

- MRI: Detects periosteal and bone marrow edema in early stress fractures.
- Radiography: Negative early; shows periosteal reaction after 2–4 weeks.
- CT: Clarifies complex fractures for surgical planning.

Key Teaching Points:

- Suspect stress fractures in musicians with persistent bone pain.
- MRI detects early edema when radiographs are negative.
- High-risk fractures require prolonged immobilization or surgery.
- CT aids pre-surgical planning for complex cases.

7 Lateral Malleolar Bursitis (Table 3)

The soft tissue around the ankle is thin, and the lateral and medial malleoli, which form the two pillars of the bony landmarks, are subcutaneous (Lee et al. 2017). These bony prominences, especially the lateral malleolus, are subjected to high levels of pressure while sitting cross-legged. This results in abnormal shear forces at the subcutaneous tissue, leading to the development of an adventitious bursa. This bursa may not always be symptomatic except when it gets irritated, resulting in discomfort and occasionally pain with the development of callosity and hyperpigmented skin (Fig. 4) (Avci and Sayli 2001).

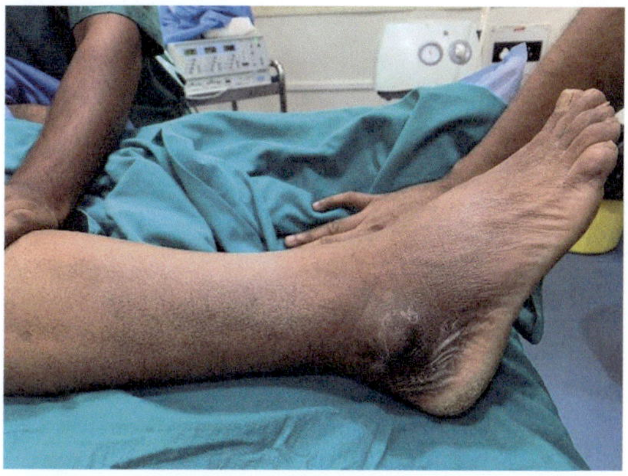

Fig. 4 Callosity with hyperpigmented skin in lateral malleolar bursitis. (Source: Author)

The recurrence of this bursa with repetitive shear stress due to prolonged, uniform cross-legged sitting, especially in Indian classical musicians, may result in infection (Fig. 5) (Brown et al. 2000).

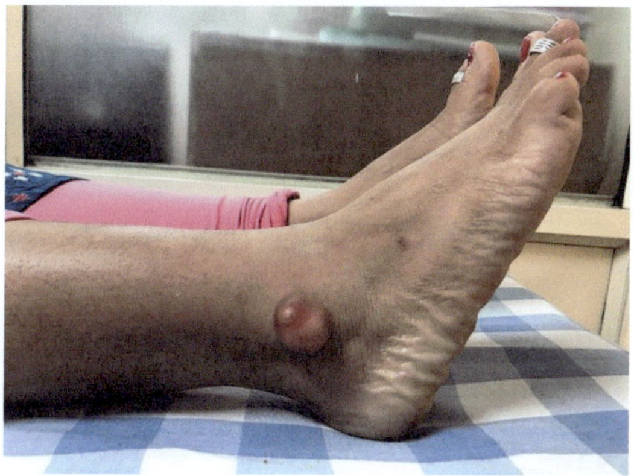

Fig. 5 Infected lateral malleolar bursitis. (Source: Author)

Aging, vascular insufficiency, and comorbidities like diabetes mellitus, as well as open wounds, will complicate healing (Hashimoto et al. 2003). This may necessitate major surgical procedures such as rotational flap coverage and prolonged recovery time (Mojallal et al. 2011).

Hence, it is mandatory to identify the risk factors such as the development of hyperpigmentation around the outer aspect of the ankle, pain while sitting cross-legged, or friction of the ankle against the floor. The presence of diabetes mellitus makes the situation worse due to delayed healing and the development of painless abscesses (Fig. 6) to non-healing ulcers, which eventually need a multidisciplinary approach including diabetic control, local dressings, excision of dead tissues, and, in some situations, plastic surgical flap coverage.

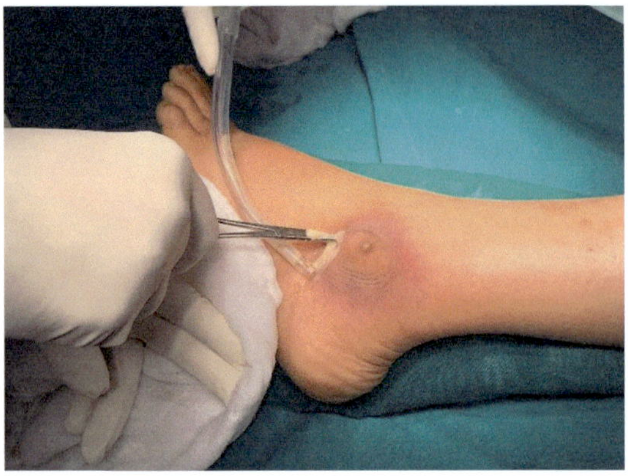

Fig. 6 Draining pus from the abscess (in a diabetic). (Source: Author)

8 Heel Pain

8.1 Plantar Fasciitis to Plantar Fasciosis

Pain in the heel, especially in the first few steps in the morning, is a typical presentation of a common cause of heel pain in middle age. With better understanding over the years, the condition is now established as degenerative in nature, in comparison to inflammation which was the earlier belief.

Plantar fascia is a thick band of fibrous connective tissue spanning from the posterior tuberosity of the calcaneum to the foot base of the proximal phalanges. It consists of a medial band which extends towards the hallux, a lateral band which extends towards the base of the 5th metatarsal, and a central band which usually gets involved in the condition. This band is thickest, strongest, and divides into five bundles at metatarsal levels, each attaching to the plantar plate of each proximal phalanx, respectively (Latt et al. 2020).

Risk factors include:

1. Obesity (BMI >30)
2. Female gender
3. Third to fourth decade of life
4. Standing for long hours
5. Pre-existing flatfoot
6. Tightness of heel cord

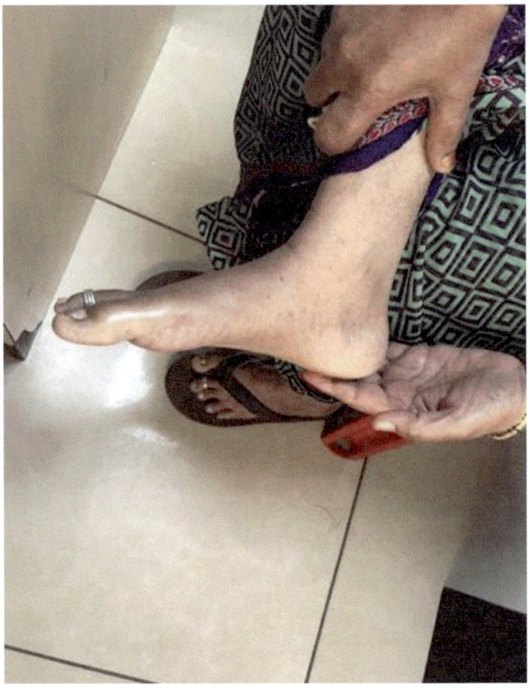

Fig. 7 Heel pain in plantar fasciitis/fasciosis. (Source: Author)

8.2 Key History

An individual complains of pain at the heel (Fig. 7) in the first few steps from the bed in the early morning, pain in the heel after prolonged standing or sitting for hours, like soon after the concert first few steps, pain at the ball of the heel.

On examination, tenderness is present at the medial calcaneal eminence and along the central band of the plantar fascia.

Dorsiflexion of the ankle, if less than 10° compared to the contralateral side, suggests heel cord tightness.

9 Investigations

- Plain radiograph: may show a calcaneal spur, but this is an incidental finding and not the cause of pain (Fig. 8).
- Ultrasonography: a rapid and cost-effective assessment; plantar fascia thickness >4.5 mm with hypoechoic areas confirms diagnosis.

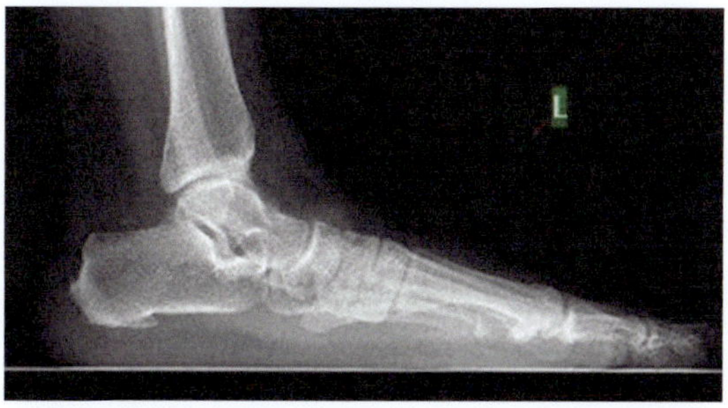

Fig. 8 Weight bearing radiograph showing Calcaneal spur, indicating chronicity of the condition. (Source: Author)

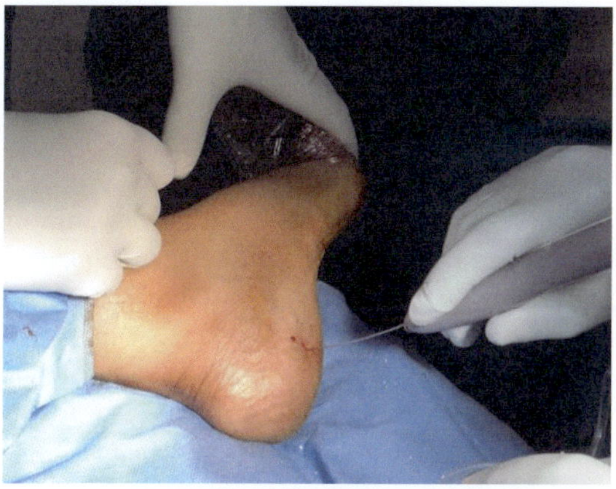

Fig. 10 Radiofrequency ablation—minimally invasive radiofrequency microablation of plantar fascia for dissolving scar tissue and stimulate neovascularization. (Source: Author)

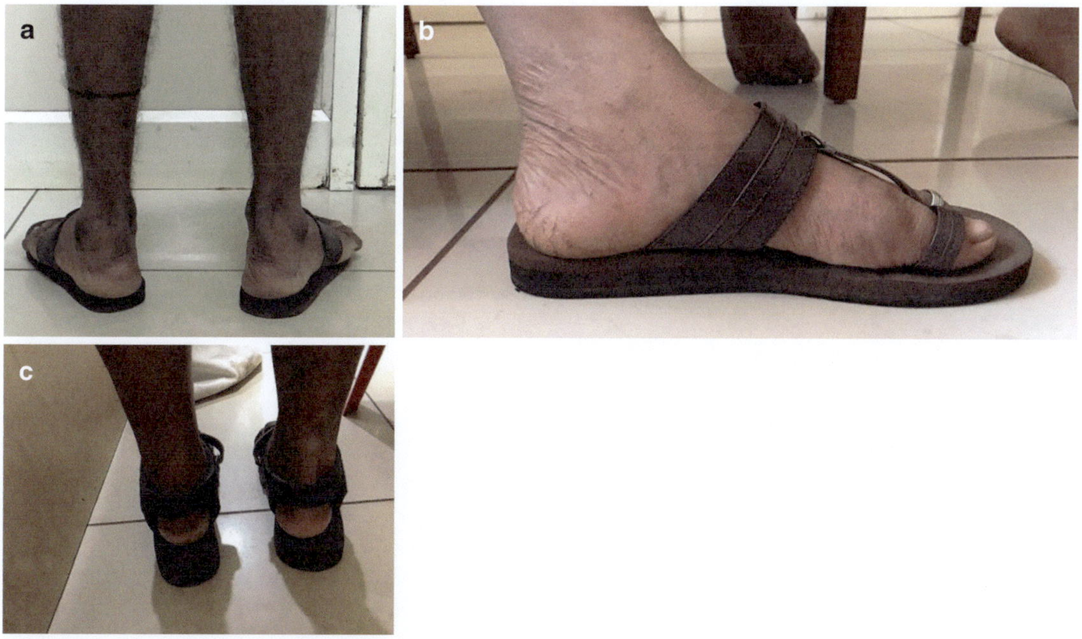

Fig. 9 (**a**–**c**): Micro Cellular Rubber (MCR) slippers with modifications. (Source: Author)

10 Management

Conservative treatment is effective in ~90% of patients and includes stretching, anti-inflammatory drugs, orthotics (Fig. 9), physical therapy, night splints, and walking casts.

Invasive options include local corticosteroid or platelet-rich plasma injections or radiofrequency microablation (Fig. 10). In resistant cases, endoscopic plantar fascia release or fasciotomy may be indicated.

11 Achilles Tendinopathy with Haglund Deformity (with or Without Tendon Rupture) (Table 3)

Achilles tendon or calf pain is a major cause of overuse injuries, often presenting as heel pain or a posterior heel "hump bump" (Haglund deformity) (Fig. 11). This occurs in younger individuals engaged in sports or in middle-aged musicians who suddenly take up recreational exercise to prevent lifestyle disorders such as obesity or diabetes, leading to aggravation of symptoms.

The Achilles tendon is formed by the gastrocnemius and soleus muscles (with plantaris), composed of type I collagen, and surrounded by paratenon which provides nutrition. With aging, collagen integrity reduces, fat infiltration and capillary proliferation occur, and partial tendon tears heal with calcium deposition, producing calcific tendinopathy (Chimenti et al. 2017). Haglund deformity (Fig. 11) occurs due to impingement of deep tendon fibers, causing chronic tendon tears.

Clinical Features

- Swelling at the back of the heel
- Tenderness at the distal tendon insertion
- Limitation of active dorsiflexion
- Inability to stand on a single heel raise
- In advanced or late presentation cases, a palpable gap suggesting rupture/tear of Achilles tendon associated with tenderness (Fig. 12).

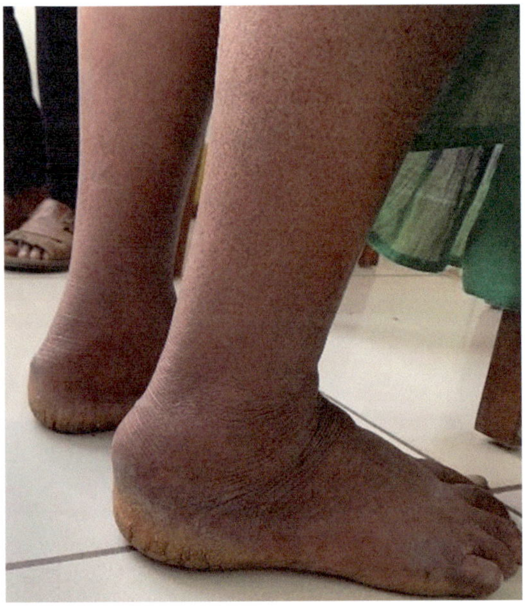

Fig. 11 Haglund deformity at the right heel. (Source: Author)

Imaging

- Radiographs: intratendinous osteophytes
- Ultrasound: diagnosis of tendinopathy or calcification
- MRI: assessment of tendon degeneration and tear extent (Fig. 13)

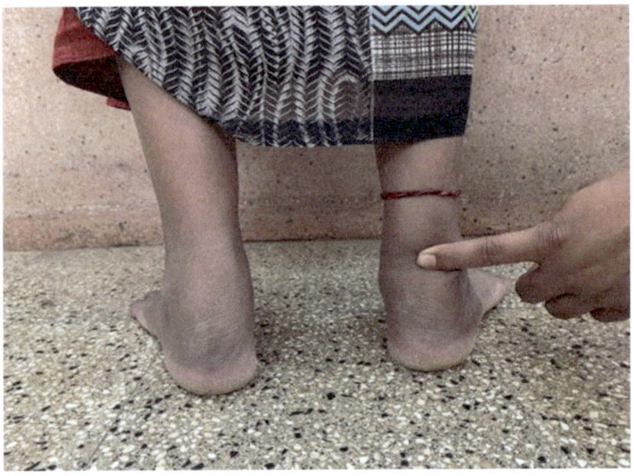

Fig. 12 Loss of normal contour of Achilles tendon with gap in the substance of the tendon. (Source: Author)

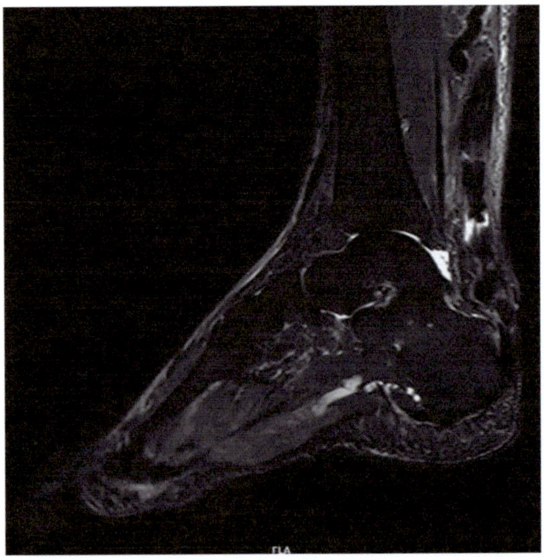

Fig. 13 MRI showing the tear and amount of segmental degeneration. (Source: Author)

12 Management

Non-operative: anti-inflammatory medication, splinting with CAM boot (Fig. 14), eccentric strengthening, extracorporeal shock wave therapy. Corticosteroid injection is avoided due to risk of iatrogenic rupture.

Operative (Fig. 15): aims at debridement of unhealthy tendon, excision of Haglund deformity, and tendon repair/augmentation. Tendon transfer may be required in chronic rupture (Feng et al. 2024).

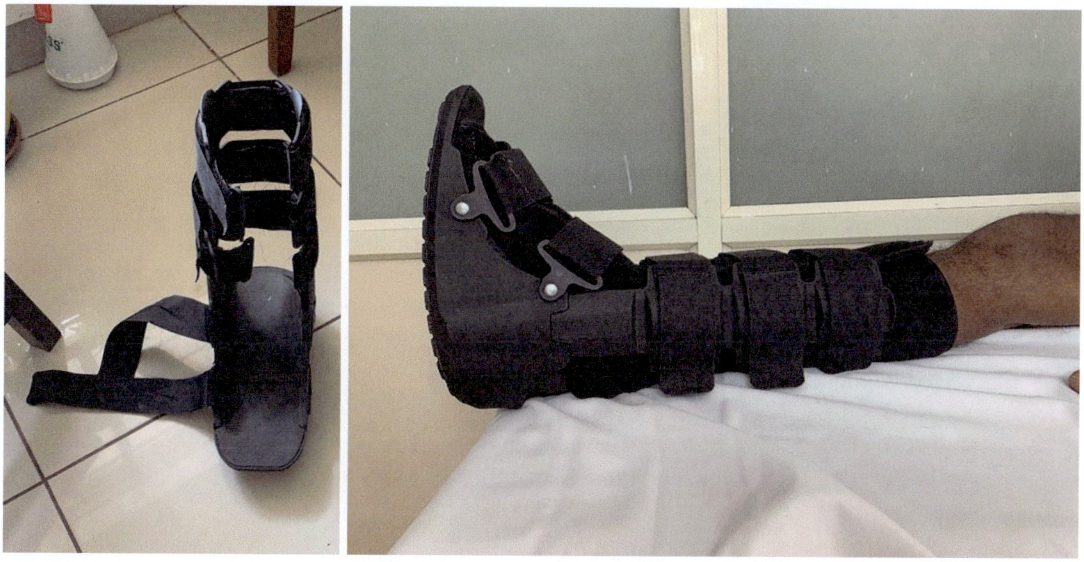

Fig. 14 CAM boot with modification-heel raise wedges. (Source: Author)

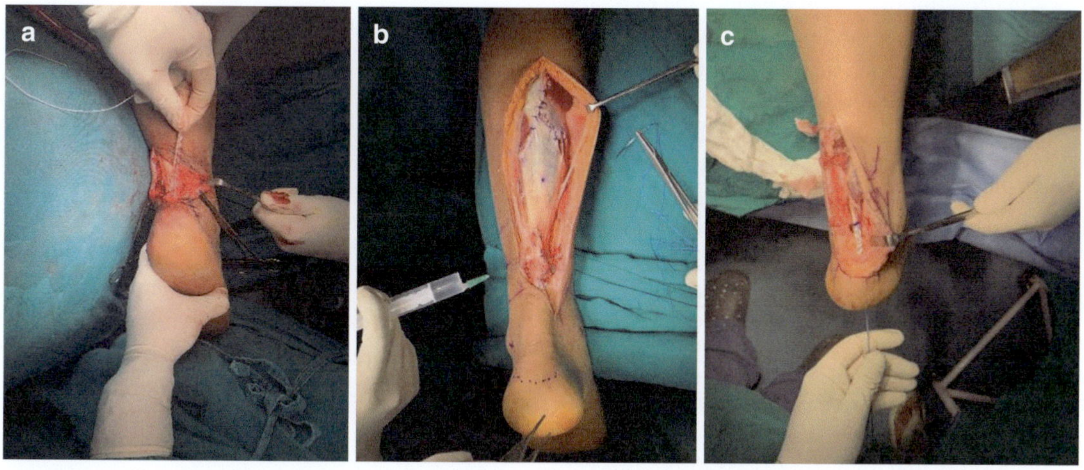

Fig. 15 (**a**) Direct repair, (**b**) V-Y plasty augmentation, (**c**) FHL tendon augmentation. (Source: Author)

Table 4 Rehabilitation protocols for ankle injuries
Rehabilitation strategies for ankle injuries in Indian classical musicians

Condition	Goals	Exercises
CPN Palsy	Prevent contracture; strengthen	AFO; passive range of motion (ROM); nerve glides; dorsiflexion/eversion.
TTS	Reduce compression; stabilize foot	Nerve glides; towel scrunches; inversion; calf stretching.
Posterior Tibialis Tendinopathy	Heal tendon; correct biomechanics	Eccentric heel drops; orthotics; hip/core strengthening.
Anterior Tibialis Tendinopathy	Reduce inflammation; strengthen	Resisted dorsiflexion; calf stretching; ankle circles.
Bone Stress Injury	Heal bone; reduce loading	Boot; cross-training; gradual tapping reintroduction.
Lateral Malleolar Bursitis	Reduce inflammation; prevent recurrence	Stretching; padded supports; core strengthening.
Achilles Tendinopathy	Heal tendon; reduce impingement	Eccentric calf exercises; Achilles of loading; stretching.

Source: Author

13 Conservative Management (Table 4)

- Activity Modification: Reduce talam intensity or cross-legged sitting. Mental practice preserves skills (Yu et al. 2013).
- Pharmacotherapy: NSAIDs reduce inflammation (Quirk 2008).
- Cryotherapy: Ice alleviates pain and swelling (Quirk 2008).
- Orthotics/Bracing: An ankle-foot orthosis (AFO) prevents foot drop in CPN palsy; arch-support orthotics reduce strain in TTS and posterior tibialis tendinopathy; walking boots immobilize stress fractures; padded inserts reduce bursal pressure; Achilles offloading braces reduce tendon strain (Chandra et al. 2017; Quirk 2008; Warden et al. 2014; Lee et al. 2017; Chimenti et al. 2017).

14 Physical Therapy (Table 4)

- Nerve Entrapments: Nerve gliding and strengthening (e.g., dorsiflexion for CPN palsy, intrinsic foot exercises for TTS) restore function (Chandra et al. 2017; Quirk 2008).
- Tendinopathies: Eccentric exercises, calf stretching, and proprioception training promote healing (Quirk 2008; Simpson and Howard 2009; Chimenti et al. 2017).
- Bursitis: Stretching and strengthening reduce shear stress; padded supports prevent recurrence (Lee et al. 2017).

15 Interventional/Surgical Management

- Injections: Corticosteroids relieve inflammation in TTS, tendinopathies, or bursitis, but risk tendon rupture or delayed healing (Quirk 2008; Lee et al. 2017).
- Surgery: Decompression treats refractory CPN palsy or TTS; tendon transfers or osteotomies correct advanced posterior tibialis tendinopathy; fixation stabilizes non-union stress fractures; bursal excision or flap coverage addresses chronic bursitis; Achilles debridement with Haglund excision or tendon repair treats severe cases (Chandra et al. 2017; Quirk 2008; Lee et al. 2017; Feng et al. 2024).

16 Prevention

16.1 Ergonomic and Behavioral Strategies

Prevention combines ergonomic and sports medicine principles, respecting cultural traditions (Stanhope et al. 2020).

- Postural Retraining: Cushions elevate hips, reducing ankle strain and bursal pressure; ergonomic chairs support neutral posture (Alsirhani et al. 2023; Lee et al. 2017).
- Practice Habits: Warm-ups (e.g., leg swings), cool-downs (e.g., calf stretches), and rest breaks prevent overuse (Quirk 2008; Chimenti et al. 2017).
- Footwear/Surfaces: Supportive shoes, padded inserts, and cushioned mats reduce impact and shear stress (Quirk 2008; Lee et al. 2017).

17 Conclusion

Clinical Vignette: A 45-year-old Carnatic violinist presents with a 2-week history of foot drop after a 3-h concert in Sukhasana posture. Examination reveals weak ankle dorsiflexion, numbness over the foot dorsum, and a positive Tinel's sign at the fibular head. Ultrasound shows CPN flattening at the fibular head; electrodiagnostics confirm neuropraxia. Treatment includes an AFO, avoidance of cross-legged sitting, and nerve gliding exercises. Symptoms resolve in 6 weeks, and the musician uses a cushion to prevent recurrence.

Indian classical musicians face unique ankle and foot PRMDs due to cross-legged sitting and talam-related repetitive loading, causing compressive neuropathies (CPN palsy, TTS), tendinopathies, stress fractures, and bursitis. A performance-focused history ensures accurate diagnosis, prioritizing peripheral over spinal etiologies (Chandra et al. 2017; Quirk 2008). Comprehensive management and prevention, targeting the kinetic chain with conservative, rehabilitative, and ergonomic strategies, support musician health while preserving cultural practices (Alsirhani et al. 2023; Stanhope et al. 2020).

References

Ahmad M, Tsang K, Mackenney PJ, Adedapo AO (2017) Tarsal tunnel syndrome: a literature review. Foot Ankle Surg 23(3):135–139. https://doi.org/10.1016/j.fas.2016.04.001

Alsirhani H, Arnold G, Wang W (2023) The biomechanical effects of cross-legged sitting on the lower limbs and the implications in rehabilitation. Appl Sci 13(6):4032. https://doi.org/10.3390/app13064032

Avci S, Sayli U (2001) Lateral premalleolar bursitis as a result of sitting on the foot. Foot Ankle Int 22(1):64–66

Brown TD, Varney TE, Micheli LJ (2000) Malleolar bursitis in figure skaters: indications for operative and non-operative treatment. Am J Sports Med 28(1):109–111

Chandra SR, Anand B, Issac TG (2017) Median and common peroneal neuropathy in coir workers of Alappuzha district, Kerala. Ann Indian Acad Neurol 20(1):23–28. https://doi.org/10.4103/0972-2327.199917

Chimenti RL, Cychosz CC, Hall MM, Phisitkul P (2017) Current concepts review update: insertional Achilles tendinopathy. Foot Ankle Int 38(10):1160–1169. https://doi.org/10.1177/1071100717723127

Feng SM, Maffulli N, Oliva F, Saxena A, Hao YF, Hua YH, Xu HL, Tao X, Xu W, Migliorini F, Ma C (2024) Surgical management of chronic Achilles tendon rupture: evidence-based guidelines. J Orthop Surg Res 19(1):132. https://doi.org/10.1186/s13018-024-04559-5

Hashimoto I, Yoshinaga R, Toda M, Nakanishi H (2003) Intractable malleolar bursitis treated with lateral calcaneal artery adipofascial flap. Br J Plast Surg 56(7):701–703

Latt LD, Jaffe DE, Tang Y, Taljanovic MS (2020) Evaluation and treatment of chronic plantar fasciitis. Foot Ankle Orthop 5(1):2473011419896763. https://doi.org/10.1177/2473011419896763

Lee YB, Kim DH, Jung JH, Park JY (2017) Chronic open infective lateral malleolus bursitis management using local rotational flap. Biomed Res Int 2017:2728092. https://doi.org/10.1155/2017/2728092

Mojallal A, Shipkov CD, Braye F, Breton P (2011) Distally based adipofascial sural flap for foot and ankle reconstruction. J Am Podiatr Med Assoc 101(1):41–48

Quirk R (2008) Posterior tibial tendon tears in dancers. Clin Sports Med 27(2):287–300. https://doi.org/10.1016/j.csm.2007.12.001

Simpson MR, Howard TM (2009) Tendinopathies of the foot and ankle. Am Fam Physician 80(10):1107–1114. Available at: https://www.aafp.org/afp/2009/1115/p1107

Stanhope J, Milanese S, Weinstein P (2020) Musculoskeletal disorders and complaints in professional musicians: a systematic review of prevalence, risk factors, and clinical treatment effects. Int Arch Occup Environ Health 93:149–187. https://doi.org/10.1007/s00420-019-01467-8

Warden SJ, Davis IS, Fredericson M (2014) Management and prevention of bone stress injuries in long-distance runners. J Orthop Sports Phys Ther 44(10):749–765. https://doi.org/10.2519/jospt.2014.5334

Yu JK, Yang JS, Kang SH, Cho YJ (2013) Clinical characteristics of peroneal nerve palsy by posture. J Korean Neurosurg Soc 53(5):269–273. https://doi.org/10.3340/jkns.2013.53.5.269

Rehabilitation of Musical Injuries

Karthikeyan P. Iyengar, Veenadhari Bhamidipaty, Anna-Maria Rennie, and Rajesh Botchu

Contents

Abstract

This document provides a comprehensive overview of musical injury rehabilitation, focusing on vocal injuries in singers and musculoskeletal disorders in instrumentalists. Vocal injuries, including nodules, polyps, Reinke's oedema, muscle tension dysphonia, and spasmodic dysphonia, result from phonotrauma or neurological factors and present with hoarseness, voice fatigue, and reduced range. Diagnosis involves laryngoscopy, stroboscopy, and acoustic assessments, with rehabilitation emphasising voice rest, speech-language pathology interventions, and in severe cases, medical or surgical treatment. For instrumentalists, playing-related musculoskeletal disorders (PRMDs) such as tendinopathies, nerve entrapment, and focal dystonia arise from repetitive strain across plucking, bowing, and blowing instruments. Rehabilitation incorporates rest, physical therapy, ergonomic adjustments, and gradual return-to-play protocols. Preventive strategies, including proper technique, posture correction, and fitness, are critical for both singers and instrumentalists. Supported by otolaryngology and performing arts medicine literature, this document underscores the efficacy of multidisciplinary, evidence-based approaches to restore function and prevent recurrence in musicians.

K. P. Iyengar
Department of Orthopaedics, Southport and Ormskirk Hospitals, Mersey and West Lancashire NHS Trust, Southport, UK

V. Bhamidipaty
Department of CSE, GITAM, Visakhapatnam, India

A.-M. Rennie
Leicester High School for Girls, Leicester, UK

R. Botchu (✉)
Department of MSK Radiology, Royal Orthopaedic Hospital, Birmingham, UK

Med Radiol Diagn Imaging (2025)

https://doi.org/10.1007/174_2025_624,
Published Online: 25 September 2025

1 Vocal Injuries in Singers

1.1 Vocal Anatomy

The vocal apparatus comprises the larynx (voice box) and associated structures. The vocal folds (true vocal cords) are paired mucosal folds stretched between the thyroid and arytenoid cartilages, vibrating at the glottis to produce sound. Intrinsic laryngeal muscles (e.g. cricothyroid, thyroarytenoid, lateral cricoarytenoid) finely adjust fold tension and position, while extrinsic muscles (e.g. sternothyroid, digastric) stabilise the larynx. Sound is powered by respiratory muscles (diaphragm, intercostals) generating subglottic pressure and shaped by supraglottic structures (epiglottis, pharynx, nasal passages). Efficient phonation requires symmetric vocal fold closure and coordinated muscle tone (Reiter et al. 2015). Dysphonia often arises when this balance is disrupted by hypertonicity, incomplete glottic closure, fold bulk changes, or lesions (Van Houtte et al. 2011).

1.2 Common Vocal Injuries

Vocal Nodules (Singer's nodes) Benign, bilateral callus-like lesions at the junction of anterior and middle thirds of the vocal folds, caused by chronic phonotrauma (e.g. repeated shouting or singing) leading to localised oedema and fibrosis (Kraimer and Husain 2019). Clinically, nodules cause hoarseness, breathiness, and voice fatigue.

Vocal Polyps Unilateral, soft, sessile, or pedunculated lesions from acute or chronic trauma, often precipitated by a single episode of vocal strain (e.g. shouting). Symptoms include hoarseness and possible diplophonia (Kraimer and Husain 2019).

Reinke's Oedema Diffuse swelling of the superficial lamina propria (Reinke's space), typically in smokers or with chronic overuse, resulting in a low-pitched, gravelly voice (Kraimer and Husain 2019).

Muscle Tension Dysphonia (MTD) A functional voice disorder characterised by excessive tension in extrinsic laryngeal muscles and supraglottal structures, compressing the larynx. The folds are usually anatomically normal. Patients report a strangled or effortful voice, pitch breaks, throat tightness, and early vocal fatigue (Van Houtte et al. 2011).

Vocal Fold Haemorrhage and Granuloma Acute phonotrauma can rupture a capillary (haemorrhage), causing sudden hoarseness. Granulomas (e.g. from laryngeal intubation or reflux) cause throat discomfort and voice change (Kraimer and Husain 2019).

Spasmodic Dysphonia (Laryngeal Dystonia) A neurological condition with involuntary spasms of laryngeal muscles (adductor or abductor type), causing intermittent breaks in phonation. Unlike MTD, it is involuntary and not solely due to muscle overuse (Reiter et al. 2015).

1.3 Clinical Presentation and Diagnosis

Affected singers present with hoarseness, decreased vocal range, voice fatigue, throat pain, or effort (Cohen et al. 2012). A detailed history should elicit voice habits, symptom onset, variability, and potential causes (e.g. shouting, infection). Perceptual assessment employs standardised scales (e.g. GRBAS or CAPE-V) to grade voice quality (Reghunathan and Bryson 2019). Physical examination may reveal neck and shoulder muscle tension.

Laryngoscopic evaluation is critical, using flexible or rigid laryngoscopy, often with stroboscopy, to visualise vocal fold vibrations. Stroboscopy identifies mucosal wave abnormalities, lesion sites, and incomplete closure (Reghunathan and Bryson 2019). For instance, nodules appear as symmetric bilateral thickenings, polyps as unilateral masses, and MTD shows excessive supraglottal compression with structurally normal folds. Imaging (CT/MRI) is rarely required unless malignancy is suspected (Steuer et al. 2017).

Diagnostic work-up includes acoustic measures and patient-reported questionnaires, such as the Voice Handicap Index, to quantify functional impact (Hogikyan and Sethuraman 1999; Rosen et al. 2004). General medical evaluation screens for reflux, allergies, thyroid disease, or neurological causes (e.g. myasthenia gravis) (Mao et al. 2001). Early referral to an otolaryngologist is recommended for persistent hoarseness exceeding 3 weeks to exclude serious pathology (Stachler et al. 2018).

1.4 Rehabilitation Protocols

Rehabilitation aims to eliminate phonotrauma and restore efficient voice production through the following:

Voice Rest and Hygiene Relative voice rest (e.g. avoiding shouting, speaking softly) is often prescribed initially, with absolute silence rarely necessary (Stachler et al. 2018). A brief period of strict rest ("vocal cool-down") can reduce acute inflammation and shrink small lesions (Kraimer and Husain 2019). Singers should maintain hydration, avoid throat clearing, and minimise irritants (e.g. smoke, reflux).

Voice Therapy with Speech-Language Pathologist (SLP) SLPs or singing therapists guide therapy to retrain breathing and phonation techniques. Methods include diaphragmatic breathing exercises, resonant voice therapy (promoting forward tone), and semi-occluded vocal tract exercises (e.g. straw phonation, lip trills) to balance subglottic pressure and glottic closure. Therapy fosters healthy voicing habits, relaxation of extrinsic muscles, and posture control. For MTD, SLPs emphasise open-mouth posture, neck relaxation, and coordinated breathing with phonation. Voice therapy is the cornerstone for nodules, polyps, and MTD (Van Houtte et al. 2011; Stachler et al. 2018).

Physical Exercises Adjunctive exercises enhance support and flexibility. Breathing exercises (e.g. sustained /s/ sounds, controlled breathflow) improve glottal efficiency. Neck and shoulder stretches (e.g. sternocleidomastoid, trapezius) alleviate ancillary tension. Combining voice exercises with postural and balance training significantly improves MTD symptoms (Van Houtte et al. 2011). Postural control techniques (e.g. Alexander technique elements) and shoulder relaxation are often incorporated.

Medical and Surgical Interventions (if needed) Short-term corticosteroids may address acute haemorrhage or severe oedema (Kraimer and Husain 2019). Microlaryngoscopic excision is reserved for large polyps, cysts, or persistent nodules after conservative measures. Post-surgical voice therapy and rest are essential for optimal healing (Francis and Smith 2019).

Evidence supports this approach, with studies showing that voice rest and steroids reduce lesion size in most singers with vocal fold trauma (Kraimer and Husain 2019). The American Academy of Otolaryngology–Head and Neck Surgery (AAO-HNS) guideline advocates early intervention and voice therapy to restore phonation (Stachler et al. 2018). Up to 80%–90% of vocal nodules resolve with therapy alone, and prolonged voice rest, beyond a few days, offers no additional benefit over guided therapy (Francis and Smith 2019). Rehabilitation significantly improves voice quality, with objective measures (e.g. Maximum Phonation Time, GRBAS scores) showing progress post-therapy (Van Houtte et al. 2011).

2 Instrumentalist Injuries

Instrumental musicians frequently experience playing-related musculoskeletal disorders (PRMDs) due to repetitive stress, including tendon overload, nerve entrapment, muscle strains, and postural syndromes. Management emphasises prevention (e.g. proper technique, breaks, fitness) and tailored rehabilitation (e.g. therapeutic exercises, ergonomics). Gradual return-to-play, cross-training, and healthy practice habits are essential across all instruments.

2.1 Plucking Instruments (Guitar, Harp, Etc.)

2.1.1 Relevant Anatomy

Plucking demands intricate finger, hand, and arm movements.

Fingers and Hands Flexor and extensor tendons (e.g. flexor digitorum profundus/superficialis, extensor digitorum) control finger movement, with thumb and thenar muscles critical for plectrum use and string pressure.

Wrist and Forearm The wrist (carpal bones, ligaments) and forearm muscles (wrist flexors/extensors, pronators/supinators) stabilise fine movements.

Elbow and Arm Repetitive finger motion and hand positioning stress the elbow (e.g. lateral epicondyle), with upper-arm muscles (biceps/triceps) supporting instrument positioning.

Shoulder and Neck Holding a guitar or harp tensions the shoulder (supraspinatus, trapezius) and cervical spine, particularly with poor posture.

2.1.2 Common Injuries (Table 1)

Tendinopathies Overuse of finger or wrist tendons causes tendinitis/tenosynovitis. De Quervain's tenosynovitis (thumb tendon sheath) is common in guitarists with heavy picking, while finger flexor tenosynovitis (trigger finger) and wrist extensor/flexor tendinitis arise from sustained postures.

Nerve Entrapments Repetitive flexion/extension compresses nerves, leading to carpal tunnel syndrome (median nerve at wrist, causing numbness in thumb/first two fingers), Guyon's canal syndrome (ulnar nerve at wrist), cubital tunnel syndrome (ulnar nerve at elbow), or radial tunnel syndrome (posterior interosseous nerve, causing forearm pain).

Table 1 Plucking instruments

Common injuries	Rehabilitation approach	Red flags
De Quervain's tenosynovitis, trigger finger, carpal tunnel syndrome	Relative rest, thumb spica/ wrist splints, eccentric exercises, ergonomic adjustments (e.g. lighter picks)	Persistent numbness (neuropathy), involuntary finger contractions (focal dystonia)
Wrist tendinitis, osteoarthritis	Stretching, strengthening, transverse friction massage, neutral wrist posture	Joint deformity, severe stiffness
Focal hand dystonia	Sensory retraining, technique modification	Task-specific cramping unresponsive to therapy

Source: Author (2025)

Joint/Overuse Syndromes Chronic strain may result in finger joint osteoarthritis (common in older guitarists) or Linburg–Comstock anomaly, a congenital flexor tendon connection causing pain between thumb and index motion.

Cramping and Dystonia Focal hand dystonia (e.g. "guitarist's cramp") is a rare, task-specific motor control disorder causing involuntary finger contractions, potentially career-threatening.

2.1.3 Diagnosis

Evaluation begins with a history of symptoms (e.g. pain location, onset with practice). Physical examination includes the following:

Provocative Tests Finkelstein's test (thumb extension with ulnar deviation) for De Quervain's; Tinel's/Phalen's for carpal tunnel; resisted wrist/finger extension for tendinitis. Grip and pinch strength are assessed.

Neurologic Exam Assesses hand sensation, motor function (e.g. finger abduction for ulnar nerve), and reflexes.

Imaging Ultrasound or MRI confirms tendon tears or joint arthritis; nerve conduction studies quantify neuropathy, particularly before surgical decompression.

Differential Diagnosis Distinguishes overuse pain from cervical radiculopathy (via neck exam) or central neurological conditions.

2.1.4 Rehabilitation Protocols (Table 1)

Rehabilitation is multidisciplinary, involving physical/occupational therapists with musician expertise:

Rest and Activity Modification Initial relative rest from aggravating activities is advised, avoiding prolonged practice without breaks (e.g. 10–15-min breaks hourly). Patients are educated on the "stop principle", ceasing activity at the onset of pain to prevent exacerbation.

Immobilisation/Splinting Short-term splints offload injured tendons or nerves (e.g. thumb spica splint for De Quervain's, neutral-position wrist splints for carpal tunnel), typically for weeks to facilitate healing.

Physical Therapy Emphasises gentle stretching of forearm/wrist muscles and strengthening of intrinsic hand muscles. Eccentric exercises (e.g. slow finger extension against resistance) target tendinopathies. Techniques include transverse friction massage for tendon sheaths, ultrasound therapy, or heat to reduce stiffness. Tailored programs addressing core, shoulder, and neck muscles reduce PRMDs.

Ergonomic Modification Instrument and technique adjustments minimise strain. Guitarists should use a strap to maintain the neck at chest level, avoiding extreme shoulder abduction, and select lighter picks or thinner finger picks for harps. Proper hand postures (neutral wrist, curved fingers), chair height, and back support are critical. Technique lessons may promote load distribution (e.g. alternating picking).

Postural Correction Addresses neck/shoulder posture by stretching tight upper trapezius or pectoral muscles and strengthening scapular stabilisers (middle trapezius, rhomboids) and thoracic extensors for upright posture.

Neuromuscular Training For focal dystonia, sensory retraining (e.g. slowed finger movements, varied tactile cues) is employed, though evidence is limited. Botulinum toxin shows no clear benefit for musician's dystonia.

Return-to-Play Guidelines Practice resumes gradually, with 10%–20% increments of pre-injury duration/force weekly, monitored for symptoms. Employ warm-up exercises, such as gentle finger flexion/extension and tendon-gliding movements, to facilitate neuromuscular coordination and reduce injury risk. Cease activity at the onset of pain.

Most PRMDs in plucking instrumentalists resolve with rest, targeted therapy, and ergonomic changes, improving pain and function through musician-specific physiotherapy.

2.2 Bowing Instruments (Violin, Cello, Etc.)

2.2.1 Relevant Anatomy

Bowing instruments require sustained asymmetric postures.

Shoulders/Arms The bow arm (right for right-handed players) elevates and rotates the shoulder, engaging rotator cuff muscles (supraspinatus, infraspinatus), deltoid, and trapezius. The left shoulder, abducted and flexed to hold the violin under the chin, involves levator scapulae and scalene muscles.

Elbow and Forearm Pronator/supinator muscles control bow rotation, with repetitive right elbow movements predisposing to epicondylitis. The left forearm grips the neck, risking flexor strain (e.g. tommy finger) during fine fingering.

Wrist and Hand Wrists may deviate (bow wrist slightly extended, fingerboard wrist flexed/extended for position shifts).

Cervical Spine and Back Violinists' neck tilt/rotation to support the instrument strains neck extensors, potentially causing tension headaches. Asymmetric stance stresses the thoracic spine.

2.2.2 Common Injuries (Table 2)

Rotator Cuff Tendinopathy Overhead arm positioning causes supraspinatus tendinitis or impingement, particularly in older players, presenting as lateral shoulder pain and abduction weakness.

Trapezius/Levator Strain Elevated shoulders during intense playing lead to trapezius muscle knots and chronic neck/shoulder pain.

Lateral (Tennis) or Medial (Golfer's) Epicondylitis Repetitive bowing strains lateral (extensor) or medial (flexor) elbow tendons, causing tenderness and pain with resisted wrist movements.

Wrist Tendinopathy Constant bow grip risks De Quervain's or extensor carpi ulnaris tendinitis (right), while fingerboard pressure causes flexor tenosynovitis (left).

Cervicalgia and Postural Syndromes Chronic neck flexion/rotation induces cervical facet stress and myofascial pain, with some violinists developing thoracic outlet syndrome from sustained neck rotation.

Focal Hand Dystonia Rare, task-specific hand cramping (e.g. involuntary finger contractions on fingerboard).

2.2.3 Diagnosis

History/Exam Notes pain asymmetry (bow vs. finger arm). Tests include empty-can (for supraspinatus), Spurling's (for cervical roots), and range of motion assessment. Palpate forearm/wrist tendons and check Tinel's sign at elbow/wrist. Inspect head carriage and scapular posture.

Imaging/Studies Ultrasound or MRI for rotator cuff tears; X-rays for arthritis; EMG/nerve conduction studies for suspected neuropathy (e.g. cervical radiculopathy, thoracic outlet syndrome).

2.2.4 Rehabilitation Protocols (Table 2)

Posture Retraining Ensures ergonomic positioning. Violinists adjust chinrest/shoulder rests to minimise neck tilt, keeping shoulders relaxed. Cellists adjust endpin height and use straps for upright posture.

Strength and Flexibility Scapular stabilisation (rows, scapular retractions) strengthens mid-back; pectoralis major and upper trapezius stretches improve flexibility; rotator cuff

Table 2 Bowing instruments

Common injuries	Rehabilitation approach	Red flags
Rotator cuff tendinopathy, epicondylitis	Scapular stabilisation, eccentric exercises, adjusted chinrest/endpin, loose bow grip	Persistent shoulder weakness, elbow locking
Trapezius strain, cervicalgia	Neck/shoulder stretches, massage, neutral neck posture	Numbness/tingling (thoracic outlet), severe headaches
Focal hand dystonia	Sensory retraining, technique modification	Progressive movement loss, unresponsive cramping

Source: Author (2025)

strengthening (e.g. theraband external rotations); and eccentric wrist/elbow exercises balance muscle groups.

Manual Therapy Massage or trigger-point release for trapezius/levator muscles and joint mobilisations address shoulder/cervical stiffness.

Ergonomic Adjustments Optimise chin/shoulder rest comfort and cello neck support. Loose bow grip with thumb opposition reduces elbow stress; lighter bows or modified grip techniques lessen load.

Gradual Loading Reintroduce playing with warm-ups (scales, long tones) and limited practice time, using rest intervals. Apply ice/heat post-practice for pain management.

Cross-Training Cardiovascular and core exercises stabilise spine during asymmetric postures, reducing playing-related pain.

Shoulder or arm pain in violinists/cellists typically improves with technique correction, postural adjustments, and targeted exercises.

2.3 Blowing Instruments (Woodwinds and Brass)

2.3.1 Relevant Anatomy

Wind and brass performance engage the following:

Respiratory System Diaphragm and intercostal muscles generate breath pressure, with diaphragmatic breathing sustaining high intraoral pressure. Core strength (abdominals, lumbar muscles) supports posture.

Lips and Face (Embouchure) Lip muscles (orbicularis oris, buccinator) and facial muscles maintain mouthpiece seal, innervated by facial/trigeminal nerves. Teeth and jaw alignment affect embouchure.

Tongue and Jaw Tongue (hypoglossal nerve) aids articulation; TMJ and masseter muscles are strained by sustained mouthpiece pressure.

Neck and Shoulders Heavy instruments (e.g. tuba, sax) strain cervical/trapezius muscles, causing chronic neck pain.

Upper Limbs Arms (e.g. trombone slide arm, alto flute position) experience secondary stress.

2.3.2 Common Injuries (Table 3)

Embouchure Dystonia Task-specific focal dystonia of lip/tongue muscles, causing loss of pitch control or involuntary movements during play, challenging to treat.

TMJ Syndrome/Facial Pain Bruxism/clenching against mouthpiece causes jaw pain, clicking, or dental issues.

Stress Velopharyngeal Incompetence (SVPI) Air leakage through soft palate in high-pressure playing (e.g. clarinet, saxophone), causing nasal tone or high-note difficulty, diagnosed via nasopharyngoscopy.

Table 3 Blowing instruments

Common injuries	Rehabilitation approach	Red flags
Embouchure dystonia, TMJ syndrome	Soft mouthpiece, dental splints, TMJ stretches, breathing exercises	Loss of pitch control, persistent jaw clicking
Stress velopharyngeal incompetence, breathing-related strain	Diaphragmatic breathing training, posture correction	Nasal air escape, progressive dyspnoea
De Quervain's, thoracic outlet syndrome	Wrist supports, shoulder relaxation, ergonomic adjustments	Persistent numbness, tingling in arms

Source: Author (2025)

Breathing-Related Rare diaphragmatic/intercostal strain or lower back pain from overuse; asthma patients may experience exercise-induced bronchoconstriction (Ishizuka et al. 2007).

Other Musculoskeletal Tendonitis (e.g. De Quervain's in flute players) or thoracic outlet syndrome (oboe players elevating shoulders).

2.3.3 Diagnosis

Embouchure Issues Neurological exam for facial nerve; EMG in specialised centres for dystonia; dental exam for alignment; nasopharyngoscopy for SVPI.

Respiratory Assessment Spirometry for shortness of breath (Ishizuka et al. 2007); observe breathing technique.

Musculoskeletal Exam Palpate lip/jaw/neck muscles; assess shoulder range of motion.

2.3.4 Rehabilitation Protocols (Table 3)

Breathing and Core Training Diaphragmatic inhalation/exhalation exercises (e.g. sustained hisses, straw phonation) enhance stamina; core/lumbar strengthening stabilises breathing. Postural exercises improve outcomes, as seen in MTD (Van Houtte et al. 2011).

Embouchure Retraining Use soft mouthpieces, low-volume long tones, or adjusted lip/reed positions; dental splints may aid dystonia. Focus on gentle retraining with altered fingerings or key sizes.

Postural Adjustments Optimise brass mouthpiece size and tuba harness; keep woodwind elbows low; maintain relaxed, neutral neck/shoulders with breaks.

TMJ/Oral Care Dental consults for bite guards; TMJ stretches (gentle jaw opening, controlled chewing) reduce pain.

Physical Therapy Cervical/trapezius stretches, scapular strengthening prevent slouching.

Ergonomics Use neck strap pads (saxophone), wrist supports (flute), and optimised mouthpiece angles.

Gradual Practice and Rest Warm up with middle-register notes, take frequent breaths, and rest (50 min on, 10 off). Cease activity at pain onset.

Referral to performing arts medicine specialists is often needed for embouchure issues, but general physical therapy (breathing, posture, stretches) is broadly effective.

2.3.5 Key Takeaways for Musicians

Injury prevention is critical, emphasising structured warm-ups, regular breaks, posture management, and fitness (aerobic conditioning, strength training) to mitigate PRMD risk. Performing arts specialists and physical therapists advocate education on healthy practices, tailored exercises, and ergonomic adaptations. Return-to-play should be gradual, starting at 10%–20% of usual intensity, progressing only if pain-free, ensuring sustained performance capacity.

2.3.6 Clinical Insight

Up to 90% of vocal nodules resolve with voice therapy alone, highlighting its efficacy (Stachler et al. 2018). Most PRMDs in instrumentalists improve with tailored rest, technique correction, and graded return-to-play protocols, underscoring the value of multidisciplinary rehabilitation.

References

Cohen SM, Kim J, Roy N, Asche C, Courey M (2012) Prevalence and causes of dysphonia in a large treatment-seeking population. Laryngoscope 122(2):343–348. Available at: https://doi.org/10.1002/lary.22426

Francis DO, Smith LJ (2019) Hoarseness guidelines redux: toward improved treatment of patients with dysphonia. Otolaryngol Clin N Am 52(4):597–605. Available at: https://doi.org/10.1016/j.otc.2019.03.006

Hogikyan ND, Sethuraman G (1999) Validation of an instrument to measure voice-related quality of life (V-RQOL). J Voice 13(4):557–569. Available at: https://doi.org/10.1016/S0892-1997(99)80010-1

Ishizuka T, Hisada T, Aoki H, Yanagitani N, Kaira K, Utsugi M, Shimizu Y, Sunaga N, Dobashi K, Mori M (2007) Gender and age risks for hoarseness and dysphonia with use of a dry powder fluticasone propionate inhaler in asthma. Allergy Asthma Proc 28(5):550–556. Available at: https://doi.org/10.2500/aap.2007.28.3032

Kraimer KL, Husain I (2019) Updated medical and surgical treatment for common benign laryngeal lesions. Otolaryngol Clin N Am 52(4):745–757. Available at: https://doi.org/10.1016/j.otc.2019.03.017

Mao VH, Abaza M, Spiegel JR, Mandel S, Hawkshaw M, Heuer RJ, Sataloff RT (2001) Laryngeal myasthenia gravis: report of 40 cases. J Voice 15(1):122–130. Available at: https://doi.org/10.1016/S0892-1997(01)00012-0

Reghunathan S, Bryson PC (2019) Components of voice evaluation. Otolaryngol Clin N Am 52(4):589–595. Available at: https://doi.org/10.1016/j.otc.2019.03.005

Reiter R, Hoffmann TK, Pickhard A, Brosch S (2015) Hoarseness—causes and treatments. Dtsch Arztebl Int 112(19):329–337. Available at: https://doi.org/10.3238/arztebl.2015.0329

Rosen CA, Lee AS, Osborne J, Zullo T, Murry T (2004) Development and validation of the voice handicap index-10. Laryngoscope 114(9):1549–1556. Available at: https://doi.org/10.1097/00005537-200409000-00009

Stachler RJ, Francis DO, Schwartz SR, Damask CC, Digoy GP, Krouse HJ, McCoy SJ, Ouellette DR, Patel RR, Reavis CCW, Smith LJ, Smith M, Strode SW, Woo P, Nnacheta LC (2018) Clinical practice guideline: hoarseness (dysphonia) (update). Otolaryngol Head Neck Surg 158(1_suppl):S1–S42. Available at: https://doi.org/10.1177/0194599817751030

Steuer CE, El-Deiry M, Parks JR, Higgins KA, Saba NF (2017) An update on larynx cancer. CA Cancer J Clin 67(1):31–50. Available at: https://doi.org/10.3322/caac.21386

Van Houtte E, Van Lierde K, Claeys S (2011) Pathophysiology and treatment of muscle tension dysphonia: a review of the current knowledge. J Voice 25(2):202–207. Available at: https://doi.org/10.1016/j.jvoice.2009.10.009

The Aesthetics of Music and Physical Fitness: Exploring the Interplay Among Indian Musicians

Subrahmanyam Velcheti, Akanksh Chokkapu, Siva Sai Gorle, and Kanaka Durga Prasad Bhamidipaty

Contents

Abstract

Music performance is a multisensory and embodied art form, yet the physical fitness of musicians is often overlooked in musical aesthetics. This chapter examines the interplay between music aesthetics and musicians' health among Indian classical musicians, with comparative global insights. Drawing on Indian and Western theoretical frameworks, we explore how physical and mental well-being influences artistry and performance quality. We review physiological demands on Indian musicians, prevalence of performance-related injuries, and impacts on aesthetic output, alongside gender-based biases and cognitive-emotional fitness. Ethnographic vignettes illustrate real-world challenges and strategies. This chapter advocates for interdisciplinary research and educational initiatives to support healthy, expressive musicians.

1 Introduction

Music-making is a physically and mentally demanding act, requiring breath, posture, and muscle coordination to produce sound, whether singing a Hindustani *raga* or playing intricate tabla rhythms. In Indian traditions, *naada* (sound) intertwines with bodily discipline, yet physical health has historically been secondary to

S. Velcheti
The Hindu, Visakhapatnam, India

A. Chokkapu · S. S. Gorle · K. D. P. Bhamidipaty (✉)
Department of Radiodiagnosis, NRIIMS, Visakhapatnam, India

Med Radiol Diagn Imaging (2025)
https://doi.org/10.1007/174_2025_627,

Published Online: 08 October 2025

aesthetic and spiritual concerns. Recent advances in performing arts medicine highlight musicians' athletic demands, showing that physical fitness enhances endurance, prevents injuries, and improves performance quality (Rotter et al. 2020). This chapter explores how musicians' health shapes aesthetic output among Indian classical musicians, with Western comparisons.

Key questions include the following: How does physical fitness influence musical performance quality? How do injuries affect expressivity? How do gender and body image impact musicians' careers and audience perception? We also examine cognitive and emotional fitness, critical for improvisation and emotional depth. Through ethnographic vignettes and empirical data, we bridge musicology and health sciences, addressing unique Indian practices like prolonged cross-legged postures. This chapter argues that a healthy body and mind are vital for musical excellence, filling a gap in Western-centric literature.

The Introduction outlines the topic's significance, followed by a Theoretical Background comparing Indian and Western perspectives. Physical Fitness in Indian Musicians reviews health challenges, Aesthetic Output and Musicians' Health links physicality to artistry, and Gender and Aesthetic Bias explores societal influences. Cognitive and Emotional Fitness examines mental resilience, and Ethnographic Vignettes provide real-world context. The Discussion synthesizes findings, and the Conclusion offers future directions.

2 Theoretical Background

Indian aesthetic philosophy views music as a holistic pursuit, engaging body, mind, and spirit. Texts like the *Natyashastra* and *nada yoga* link physical discipline to artistic excellence. *Nada yoga* posits that sound vibrations, combined with postures and breath, elevate spiritually. Central to Indian music is *rasa* (emotional essence), where *ragas* evoke sentiments like *shringara* (romance) or *karuna* (pathos) through precise vocal or instrumental control (Hegde 2017). This requires physical and mental absorption, akin to meditation, making the performer's health integral to aesthetic impact.

Western perspectives, emerging in the twentieth century, treat musicians as "athletes of small muscles," emphasizing muscular conditioning and injury prevention (Rotter et al. 2020). Conservatory training historically prioritized technique, but performing arts medicine now incorporates somatic methods like the Alexander Technique to reduce tension and enhance expressivity. However, Western traditions once normalized over-practice, risking injury. Recent holistic approaches align with Indian views, recognizing wellness as essential for artistry.

Indian training, rooted in the *guru–shishya* system, emphasizes immersive practice (*riyaz*), often neglecting biomedical concerns like posture. Western education, by contrast, increasingly includes wellness curricula. Indian ideals prioritize the music over the performer's body, historically evident in female vocalists' restrained stage presence to avoid objectification (Alaghband-Zadeh 2015). Both traditions now acknowledge that physical health underpins technique and expression, inviting interdisciplinary insights.

3 Physical Fitness in Indian Musicians

Indian classical musicians face unique physical demands due to prolonged cross-legged sitting (*padmasana*) and repetitive movements. A study of 35 instrumentalists found 91% reported wrist pain, 89% lower back pain, and 71% neck pain, linked to unsupported postures and fine motor tasks (Patel and Rajput 2023). Tabla players, for instance, experience 43%–50% prevalence of musculoskeletal pain, particularly in shoulders and knees, due to vigorous hand motions and folded-knee positions (Mishra et al. 2013). Vocalists face vocal fold strain, with many relying on home remedies rather than professional care (Nair et al. 2021).

Core strength is critical for postural stability, with higher BMI correlating to weaker core endurance, increasing injury risk (Patel and Rajput 2023). Yoga and *pranayama* are increasingly adopted, improving flexibility and breath control. For example, hip-opening stretches alleviate sitting-related stiffness, and breathing exercises enhance vocal stamina. Instrument-specific regimens, like wrist exercises for mridangam players, also emerge. Unlike Western music education, which formalizes wellness training, Indian training historically relies on implicit guru guidance, though modern institutions now offer health modules.

A cross-sectional study of young tabla players found 66% experienced wrist pain post-playing, underscoring the need for warm-ups and breaks (Sable and Shinde 2022). Indian performances, often lasting 2–3 h, demand marathon-like stamina. Fit musicians maintain technical clarity, while fatigue can cause pitch or rhythm lapses. Emerging research advocates treating musicians as whole-body performers, integrating sports science and physiotherapy to manage health risks.

4 Sidebox: Common Musicians' Injuries

- Wrist/Hand: 91% prevalence; linked to repetitive fingerwork (e.g., sitar, tabla) (Patel and Rajput 2023).
- Lower Back: 89%; from unsupported cross-legged postures (Patel and Rajput 2023).
- Neck/Shoulders: 71%/49%; due to instrument weight (e.g., sitar) or angles (e.g., Carnatic violin) (Patel and Rajput 2023).
- Vocal Strain: Common in singers; often untreated professionally (Nair et al. 2021).

5 Aesthetic Output and Musicians' Health

Musicians' health directly shapes aesthetic output, as artistry relies on physical execution. Pain or fatigue disrupts the "flow" state, a condition of full absorption critical for transcendent performances (Csikszentmihalyi 1990). For example, a vocalist with poor breath support struggles with long *alapanas*, affecting pitch stability, while a sitarist with shoulder stiffness may produce less fluid *meends*, diminishing *raga* expressivity. Physical fitness ensures technical precision, tone quality, and endurance, enabling consistent performances across slow *alaaps* and fast *taans*.

Posture influences stage presence and audience perception. An upright singer projects confidence, enhancing aesthetic impact, while slouching suggests disengagement. A tabla solo with crisp motions captivates visually and aurally, but visible discomfort (e.g., cramped fingers) breaks immersion. Physical health also supports emotional expressivity; pain distracts from conveying *rasa*, leading to mechanical performances. Interventions like physiotherapy can improve technique, as seen in a sitarist who, after shoulder therapy, reported cleaner *tans* and greater stamina.

Audiences subconsciously register performers' physical state. Comfortable musicians instill confidence, deepening listener immersion, while signs of strain (e.g., fidgeting) distract. Health removes impediments, allowing creativity and spontaneity to flourish, fulfilling Indian music's aesthetic goals.

6 Gender and Aesthetic Bias

6.1 Physicality and Gender Bias

Gender norms historically shaped Indian musicians' roles, with instruments like tabla deemed male domains due to perceived physical demands. Female pioneers like Anuradha Pal faced skepticism but proved capability through discipline (Pal 2018). Over-practicing to counter bias risks injury, particularly for women percussionists. Gender-specific health issues, like vocal changes from hormonal fluctuations, are under-discussed due to stigma, leaving female singers to navigate challenges alone (Nair et al. 2021).

7 Appearance and Aesthetic Pressure

Female musicians faced pressure to project respectability, adopting restrained stage presence to focus on sound over body (Alaghband-Zadeh 2015). Modern expectations, especially in Bollywood, emphasize slimness, risking unhealthy dieting that impacts stamina. Classical audiences prioritize artistry, but high-definition broadcasts increase visual scrutiny. Male musicians face less appearance pressure but may avoid health-seeking to maintain stoic personas, reflecting gendered health attitudes (Sable and Shinde 2022). Mitigating bias ensures musicians prioritize health without stigma.

8 Cognitive and Emotional Fitness

Indian music's improvisational complexity demands cognitive fitness, including memory and focus. Long-term training enhances working memory, as shown in Carnatic musicians with over 3 years' experience (Benet et al. 2022). Daily *riyaz* fosters meditative concentration, but stress or fatigue impairs performance. Memory, vital for oral repertoires, benefits from mnemonic techniques and rest.

Performance anxiety affects 16.5%–60% of musicians, with younger and female performers at higher risk (Fernholz et al. 2019). Symptoms like shaky hands or vocal quavers disrupt artistry. Coping strategies include *pranayama*, visualization, and cognitive restructuring. Emotional resilience supports *rasa* expression, channeling emotions constructively. Offstage stressors (e.g., irregular income) risk burnout, necessitating peer or professional support. Flow states, where musicians feel "music flowing through them," enhance creativity and audience connection, requiring physical and mental health (Csikszentmihalyi 1990).

9 Ethnographic Vignettes

Vignette 1: Tabla Maestro's Adaptation—Ravi, a 45-year-old Mumbai tabla player, developed wrist tendonitis from intensive *riyaz*. After a concert disruption, he adopted physiotherapy and yoga, using cushions to ease posture. His pain reduced, and his *boles* gained delicacy, showing health's artistic benefits.

Vignette 2: Vocalist's Health Shift—Meera, a 30-year-old Carnatic singer, faced vocal fatigue. Rejecting home remedies, she consulted an ENT specialist, learning efficient vocal techniques. Her endurance improved, reflecting a cultural shift toward professional care (Sable and Shinde 2022).

Vignette 3: Female Percussionist's Triumph—Nalini, a mridangam player, overcame gender bias through refined technique and fitness (e.g., tennis for strength). Choosing comfortable attire for a televised concert, she prioritized performance, earning acclaim and mentoring young girls.

Vignette 4: Overcoming Stage Fright—Arjun, a Hindustani vocalist, tackled stage fright with a performance psychologist's help, using meditation and cognitive techniques. His *alaaps* gained boldness, highlighting mental health's role in artistry.

10 Discussion

This chapter reveals musicians' health as integral to Indian classical music's aesthetics. Interdisciplinary collaboration can integrate health into training, leveraging yoga's cultural resonance and modern physiotherapy. Comparative studies with Western musicians could identify unique Indian risk factors, as global data show up to 93% PRMD prevalence (Rotter et al. 2020). Indian studies confirm posture's role (Patel and Rajput 2023; Mishra et al. 2013).

Gender bias reduction fosters diverse talent, as seen in female-led ensembles. Mental health workshops at *sabhas* could address anxiety, aligning with *riaz*'s meditative ethos (Fernholz et al. 2019). Ergonomic innovations (e.g., sitar stands) and institutional support (e.g., Sangeet Natak Akademi guidelines) can enhance longevity. Localized research on injury prevalence and interventions (e.g., yoga's efficacy) is critical for evidence-based change.

11 Conclusion

Musicians' health is not a peripheral concern but a central pillar of aesthetic excellence, directly influencing both technical precision and emotional depth in performance. To support this, integrating practices like yoga, physiotherapy, and mental health support into formal training can significantly enhance a musician's stamina, expressivity, and career longevity (Table 1). However, the field lacks sufficient localized research on the prevalence of performance-related injuries and the effectiveness of targeted interventions. Conducting such studies is crucial to inform evidence-based policies and improve training standards. Equally important is the role of institutions—music academies, festivals, and cultural bodies must take active responsibility in promoting accessible health resources and creating an environment where physical and mental well-being (Table 1) are seen as essential components of sustainable, inclusive artistry.

Table 1 Strategies for musicians' well-being

Strategy	Purpose	Examples
Postural training	Reduce strain	Cushions; Alexander Technique
Exercise	Boost stamina	Swimming; weight training
Instrument-specific drills	Prevent injury	Wrist stretches (tabla); vocal exercises
Warm-ups/ cool-downs	Prepare/ recover	Slow scales; post-performance stretches
Yoga/ pranayama	Enhance flexibility, breath	Hip stretches; anulom-vilom
Mental training	Manage anxiety	Mindfulness; visualization
Rest	Prevent burnout	Scheduled breaks; sleep
Education	Empower self-care	Health seminars; anatomy in syllabi

Source: Author (2025)

References

Alaghband-Zadeh C (2015) Sonic performativity: analysing gender in North Indian classical vocal music. Ethnomusicol Forum 24(3):349–379. https://doi.org/10.1080/17411912.2015.1082925

Benet N, Rajalakshmi K, Kumar V (2022) Impact of more than three years of Carnatic music training on the working memory. Hear Balance Commun 20(1):8–14. https://doi.org/10.1080/21695717.2021.1943782

Csikszentmihalyi M (1990) Flow: the psychology of optimal experience. Harper & Row, New York

Fernholz I, Mumm JLM, Plag J, Noeres K, Rotter G, Willich SN et al (2019) Performance anxiety in professional musicians: a systematic review on prevalence, risk factors and clinical treatment effects. Psychol Med 49(14):2287–2306. https://doi.org/10.1017/S0033291719001910

Hegde S (2017) Music therapy for mental disorder and mental health: the untapped potential of Indian classical music. BJPsych Int 14(2):31–33. https://doi.org/10.1192/s2056474000001732

Mishra W, De A, Gangopadhyay S, Chandra AM (2013) Playing-related musculoskeletal disorders among Indian tabla players. Med Probl Perform Art 28(2):107–111. https://doi.org/10.21091/mppa.2013.2019

Nair RM, Joshi A, Gunjawate DR (2021) Knowledge, attitude and practices towards vocal health care amongst Indian Carnatic singers. J Voice [Preprint]. https://doi.org/10.1016/j.jvoice.2021.07.004

Pal A (2018) Breaking barriers: a female tabla virtuoso's journey. Sangeet Kala Vihar 45(3):22–25

Patel NPP, Rajput DA (2023) Prevalence of musculoskeletal disorder and correlation with core endurance, body mass index among Indian classical musical instrument players. Int J Multidiscip Res 5(4). https://doi.org/10.36948/ijfmr.2023.v05i04.5333

Rotter G, Muckenhuber J, Schütz M, Reibnegger G, Novak M, Weiss EM (2020) Musculoskeletal disorders and complaints in professional musicians: a systematic review of prevalence, risk factors, and clinical treatment effects. Int Arch Occup Environ Health 93(2):149–187. https://doi.org/10.1007/s00420-019-01467-8

Sable NA, Shinde N (2022) Prevalence of wrist pain in young tabla players: observational study. Int J Health Sci Res 12(5):10–14. https://doi.org/10.52403/ijhsr.20220502

Embodied Aesthetics: How Physical Vitality Shapes Musical Experience in the Western Tradition

Subrahmanyam Velcheti, Akanksh Chokkapu, Siva Sai Gorle, and Kanaka Durga Prasad Bhamidipaty

Contents

Abstract

This chapter explores the intricate relationship between physical vitality and musical aesthetics in the Western tradition, emphasizing the embodied nature of musical experience. It traces the historical evolution of Western musical thought, from ancient Pythagorean-Platonic theories linking music to cosmic and moral harmony, through Enlightenment formalism and Romantic expressivism, to contemporary frameworks of embodied cognition. This chapter examines how physical fitness influences musical preferences, with empirical evidence indicating that physically fit individuals gravitate toward high-arousal, rhythmically intense music and utilize music to enhance exercise performance. Drawing on phenomenological insights, particularly Merleau-Ponty's concept of the habitual body, and neuro-aesthetic research, it argues that music perception is a corporeal act, resonating through bodily sensations and movements. Philosophical perspectives from Kant, Schopenhauer, and modern enactive theories further illuminate how music engages the body as much as the mind. This chapter concludes that physical vitality amplifies aesthetic engagement, positioning the body as a central locus of musical experience, thus enriching our understanding of musical beauty and pleasure as somatic phenomena.

S. Velcheti
The Hindu, Visakhapatnam, India

A. Chokkapu · S. S. Gorle · K. D. P. Bhamidipaty (✉)
Department of Radiodiagnosis, NRIIMS, Visakhapatnam, India

Med Radiol Diagn Imaging (2025)
https://doi.org/10.1007/174_2025_628,
Published Online: 08 October 2025

1 Introduction

The interplay between music and the human body has long captivated scholars in Western musicology. Recent scholarship has increasingly explored how physical vitality—defined as robust health and bodily well-being—shapes aesthetic engagement with music. This chapter examines the historical evolution of Western musical aesthetics, from ancient cosmic and moral theories to Enlightenment formalism, Romantic expressivism, and contemporary embodied cognition. It investigates how physical fitness influences music appreciation, supported by empirical findings that physically fit individuals often prefer high-arousal or rhythmically intense music (Warrenburg and Huron 2019) and use music to enhance exercise performance (Ballmann 2021). Central to this discussion is the concept of embodiment: modern theories, from phenomenology to cognitive science, emphasize that musical perception is inherently corporeal, not merely cerebral. Music induces bodily sensations—upbeat rhythms may resonate in the limbs, while slower melodies are felt in the chest—suggesting that physical state modulates aesthetic response. Philosophical frameworks, including Kant's formalism, Schopenhauer's metaphysics, and Merleau-Ponty's phenomenology, are reconsidered through the lens of corporeality. Empirical musicology and neuroscience further reveal that music can rekindle bodily and psychological vitality, fostering what Martyn Evans terms "bodily fluency and vitality" (Evans 2016). This chapter argues that musical beauty and pleasure are somatic as well as mental phenomena, particularly amplified in physically fit individuals.

2 Historical Background: Music and the Body in Western Aesthetics

In ancient and medieval Western thought, music was understood through mathematical and moral frameworks. The Pythagorean-Platonic tradition equated musical harmony with cosmic order, attributing to music the power to align the soul and balance bodily humors. Plato argued that music shapes the soul's character, while Aristotle advocated its use, alongside dance, for moral education and catharsis. In the Middle Ages, music, as part of the quadrivium, was believed to influence listeners' temperaments through church modes.

Renaissance humanists reemphasized music's affective and therapeutic potential. Marsilio Ficino wrote, "I often resort to the solemn sound of the lyre and to singing to raise the mind to the highest considerations and to God" (Ficino, 1489, cited in Tomlinson 1993, p. 145), highlighting music's capacity to elevate both spirit and body. These early perspectives linked music to physical-emotional states, such as joy or sorrow, as pathways to higher understanding.

During the Enlightenment, aesthetics became more philosophical. Alexander Baumgarten defined aesthetics as the science of sensory perception (Baumgarten 1735), and Immanuel Kant posited that music's beauty stems from pure form, lacking conceptual depth, rendering instrumental music "beautiful but trivial" (Kant 1790). Kant viewed music as a sensuous pleasure, less cognitively engaging than poetry or painting, requiring words (as in opera) to fully engage the intellect.

Kant's formalism was challenged by Romantic thinkers who reintroduced the body and emotion into the aesthetic domain. Arthur Schopenhauer argued that music directly expresses the metaphysical "will," bypassing intellect to connect with existence itself (Schopenhauer 1819). This gave music a visceral, immediate quality, explaining its profound emotional impact. Later Romantics, such as Nietzsche and Wagner, celebrated music's kinship with dance and bodily movement, laying the groundwork for twentieth-century theories. By the twenty-first century, embodied cognition reframed music as action, movement, and resonance, moving beyond disembodied formalism.

3 Physical Fitness and Musical Appreciation

Contemporary research explores how physical vitality correlates with musical preferences and effects. Physically fit individuals frequently inte-

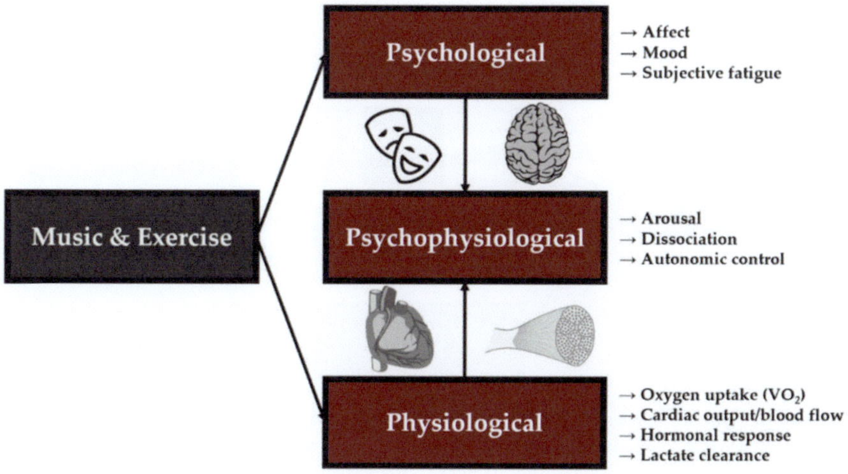

Fig. 1 Three primary areas music has been suggested to have the largest impact on are as follows: psychological, physiological, and psychophysiological. Selected variables by which music alters the experience response are shown although this is not an exhaustive list. Ultimately, psychological and physiological factors influence one another, creating an interrelated archetype for changes during exercise while listening to music (Ballmann 2021)

grate music into exercise routines (Fig. 1) (Ballmann 2021), leveraging its ability to enhance performance. Empirical studies demonstrate that music during endurance, sprint, or resistance exercise improves performance by reducing perceived exertion, increasing synchronization (e.g., running to a beat), and boosting motivation (Ballmann 2021). This creates a positive feedback loop: high-arousal (Fig. 1) (Ballmann 2021), music makes exercise more enjoyable, encouraging physical activity, which in turn heightens musical engagement.

Physically fit listeners often prefer high-arousal or rhythmically intense music, as evidenced by Warrenburg and Huron (2019), who found that individuals with higher fitness levels gravitate toward music with greater tempo, loudness, and rhythmic drive. This suggests that physical vitality expands one's aesthetic palette toward vigorous sounds. Additionally, music fosters "bodily and psychological fluency and vitality" (Evans 2016, p. 2045). Martyn Evans notes that music therapeutically rekindles embodied experience, enhancing vitality in healthy individuals.

Using earphones to enjoy music during exercise, illustrates the synergy between physical vitality and musical engagement. Controlled studies confirm that self-selected music during exercise increases motivation, reduces fatigue, and improves performance outcomes (Fig. 2) (Ballmann 2021; Thakare et al. 2017). This synergy reflects contemporary fitness culture, where music is integral to running and gym routines.

Cross-cultural research further supports these findings. Putkinen et al. (2024) found that music-induced emotions produce consistent bodily sensations across Western and Asian listeners: happy, danceable music is felt in the arms and legs, while sad, tender music resonates in the chest. These universal "bodily maps" suggest that physically fit individuals, with heightened kinesthetic awareness, may experience music's rhythms and pulses more vividly, reinforcing aesthetic engagement.

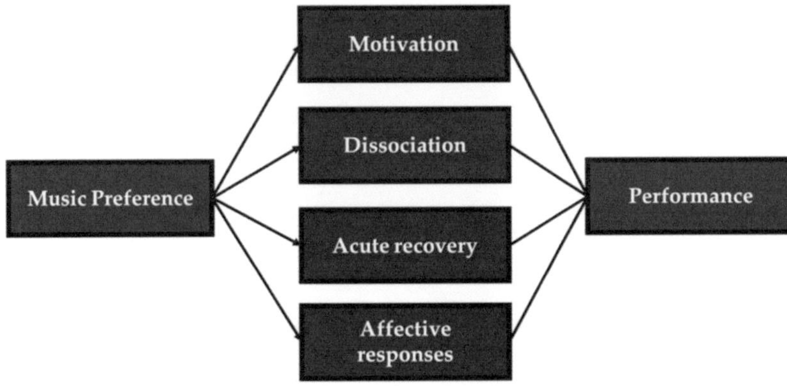

Fig. 2 The majority of evidence has suggested that music preference influences exercise performance via the following mechanisms: motivation, dissociation (lower RPE), acute recovery, and affective responses. Interactions between both psychological and physiological mechanisms are responsible for ergogenic effects. Furthermore, preferred and non-preferred music may mediate performance through a single factor listed above or through multiple mechanisms which complement one another (Ballmann 2021; Thakare et al. 2017)

4 Embodiment in Musical Experience

Embodied cognition posits that musical perception is inherently tied to the body's sensory and motor systems. Leman and Maes (2015) demonstrate that listeners' bodily movements mirror a piece's expressive qualities, with these movements shaping judgments of musical character. Musical perception engages neural circuits that prepare the body for action, encoding expressivity in motor-intentional terms. Pelinski (2005) argues that musical meaning arises from pre-rational elements like motor habits and body schemas, with rhythm and melody eliciting spontaneous bodily responses (e.g., tapping or nodding) that feed into aesthetic experience.

Phenomenologically, music reveals what Merleau-Ponty terms the "habitual body"—the structured field of perceptual engagement (Merleau-Ponty 1945). As he writes, "the body is to be compared, not to a physical object, but rather to a work of art" (Merleau-Ponty 1945, p. 150). Music expands or stabilizes this habitual body, enabling listeners to feel new motions or affirm corporeal identity (Elliott 2019). Listening is thus a corporeal act, with the body resonating with sound, blurring the line between hearing and feeling. This explains spontaneous responses like dancing or clapping, which are central to musical meaning and enjoyment.

Neuro-aesthetic research complements these insights, suggesting that mirror neurons facilitate empathetic responses to musical gestures, such as a melody evoking running feet activating gait-related neural patterns (Koelsch 2014). The "4E" cognition framework (Embodied, Embedded, Enactive, Extended) further underscores that music listening is a dynamic interaction with the environment, shaped by bodily affordances (Gallagher 2018).

5 Phenomenology and Listener Reception

Field studies of live concert audiences reveal listening as an active, embodied process. Martin and Nielsen (2024) analyzed string quartet audiences, finding that even apparent stillness involves subtle micro-movements synchronized with musical gestures. These "stilling moments" reflect kinaesthetic attunement, with listeners physically mirroring performers' phrasing. Putkinen et al. (2024) confirm that music evokes shared bodily sensations across cultures, with synchronized movements signifying social bonding. Listeners describe music in somatic terms "warm," "uplifting," or "grounding"—and report physiological changes (e.g., goosebumps, heart rate shifts) during emotional peaks, tying aesthetics to physicality.

These findings align with phenomenological accounts. Philosophers like Susanne Langer note that aesthetic experience involves a felt sense, while neuro-aesthetics highlights how synchronized movement enhances memory and social connection (Koelsch 2014). Thus, music perception, even in formal concert settings, is a full-body event, particularly pronounced in physically fit listeners with intact kinesthetic awareness.

6 Philosophical Frameworks on Music and the Body

Immanuel Kant viewed music as a sensuous pleasure, prioritizing formal beauty over conceptual depth, arguing that instrumental music requires words to engage reason fully (Kant 1790). Arthur Schopenhauer countered that music expresses the metaphysical will, connecting directly to the listener's primal drives (Schopenhauer 1819). Maurice Merleau-Ponty offered a phenomenological perspective, treating the body as the subject of perception and music as a gestural, temporal experience that reveals the habitual body (Merleau-Ponty 1945). Contemporary embodied cognition, including Gallagher's enactive-affordance perspective, views music listening as a navigation of action possibilities, grounded in sensorimotor activity (Gallagher 2018).

7 Key Philosophical Approaches (Summary)

- Kantian Formalism: Music as pure form and sensuous pleasure, lacking intrinsic meaning without textual context (Kant 1790).
- Schopenhauerian Will: Music as a direct expression of metaphysical will, penetrating beyond intellect (Schopenhauer 1819).
- Phenomenology (Merleau-Ponty): Music as embodied gesture, revealing the habitual body through kinaesthetic presence (Merleau-Ponty 1945).
- Contemporary Embodied Cognition: Music perception arises from sensorimotor activity, shaped by body and environment (Gallagher 2018).

These frameworks highlight the body's role in musical aesthetics, particularly for physically fit individuals attuned to movement and responsiveness.

8 Empirical and Musicological Research Findings

Neuroimaging studies show that rhythmic music activates motor regions (e.g., premotor cortex, basal ganglia) even in still listeners (Koelsch 2014). Warrenburg and Huron (2019) found that physical fitness predicts preferences for high-arousal music, using regression models to link fitness levels with musical intensity. Cross-cultural studies, such as Putkinen et al. (2024), confirm universal bodily sensation mappings, with rhythm and dissonance evoking innate responses. Developmental research shows infants and toddlers naturally move to music, reflecting early embodiment, while adults with higher interoceptive awareness report more intense musical experiences (Koelsch 2014).

Compositional practices also reflect embodiment, from Baroque dance suites to jazz's percussive rhythms. Performers' expressiveness relies on bodily precision (e.g., breath control in singing), and music therapy leverages movement to enhance enjoyment, supporting Evans' claim that music rekindles embodied vitality (Evans 2016). These findings underscore the inseparable link between physical condition and musical aesthetics.

9 Conclusion

Western musical thought has evolved from abstract theories to a holistic recognition of music's embodied nature. From Plato's moral harmonies to Kant's formalism, historical perspectives acknowledged music's power to move the body and soul. Modern scholarship, supported by empirical and phenomenological evidence, confirms that physically fit individuals experience music as a lived expression of vitality, amplified by their bodily attunement (Warrenburg and Huron 2019; Ballmann 2021). Music not only enhances exercise performance but also sensitizes listeners to its affective potentials, fostering a dynamic interplay of sound and movement (Ballmann 2021). Embodiment theories reveal that music is perceived through the entire body, resonating in muscles and heart as much as in the ear (Merleau-Ponty 1945). By foregrounding the somatic dimension of music, we not only expand aesthetic theory but also reconnect with the lived, moving body as the true site of musical experience.

References

Ballmann CG (2021) The influence of music preference on exercise responses and performance: a review. J Funct Morphol Kinesiol 6(2):33. Available at: https://doi.org/10.3390/jfmk6020033

Baumgarten AG (1735) Meditationes philosophicae de nonnullis ad poema pertinentibus. Hemmerde, Halle

Elliott R (2019) Collaborative temporality: Merleau-Ponty and the phenomenology of music. J Phenomenol Psychol 50(2):184–206. Available at: https://doi.org/10.1163/15691624-12341372

Evans M (2016) Music and the body: philosophical and therapeutic perspectives. Lancet 388(10055):2045–2046

Gallagher S (2018) Enactivist interventions: rethinking the mind. Oxford University Press, Oxford

Kant I (1790) Critique of judgment. Translated by W.S. Pluhar, 1987. Hackett Publishing, Indianapolis

Koelsch S (2014) Brain correlates of music-evoked emotions. Nat Rev Neurosci 15(3):170–180. Available at: https://doi.org/10.1038/nrn3666

Leman M, Maes PJ (2015) The role of embodiment in the perception of music. Empir Musicol Rev 10(3):236–246

Martin R, Nielsen N (2024) Enacting musical aesthetics: the embodied experience of live music. Music Sci 7. Available at: https://doi.org/10.1177/20592043231225732

Merleau-Ponty M (1945) Phenomenology of perception. Translated by C. Smith, 1962. Routledge, London

Pelinski R (2005) Embodiment and musical experience. Transcult Music Rev 9:1–15

Putkinen V et al (2024) Bodily maps of musical emotions across cultures. Proc Natl Acad Sci 121(5):e231170611. Available at: https://doi.org/10.1073/pnas.231170611

Schopenhauer A (1819) The world as will and representation. Translated by E.F.J. Payne, 1958. Dover Publications, New York

Thakare AE, Mehrotra R, Singh A (2017) Effect of music tempo on exercise performance and heart rate among young adults. Int J Physiol Pathophysiol Pharmacol 9(2):35–39. PMID: 28533890; PMCID: PMC5435671

Tomlinson G (1993) Music in Renaissance magic. University of Chicago Press, Chicago

Warrenburg L, Huron D (2019) Fitness and musical taste: do physically fit listeners prefer more stressful music? Empir Musicol Rev 13(1–2):21–38. Available at: https://doi.org/10.18061/emr.v13i1-2.6208

The Role of Interventional Radiology for Musicians

Neel R. Raja, Olivia Baker, Monica Hingorani, Amil Raja, Nirmal Rajagopalan, and Rajesh Botchu

Contents

N. R. Raja (✉)
Department of Radiology, Leicester Royal Infirmary, Leicester, UK

Department of Musculoskeletal Radiology, Royal Orthopaedic Hospital, Northfield, Birmingham, UK
e-mail: neelraja@doctors.org.uk

O. Baker
Ibstock & Barlestone Surgeries, Ibstock, UK

M. Hingorani
Independent Musician, De Montfort University, Leicester, UK

A. Raja
Music Producer, London, UK

N. Rajagopalan
Independent Musician, Leicester, UK

R. Botchu
Department of Musculoskeletal Radiology, Royal Orthopaedic Hospital, Northfield, Birmingham, UK

Abstract

Playing-related musculoskeletal (MSK) disorders are prevalent among musicians due to the repetitive and demanding nature of instrumental performance. Interventional radiology offers a patient-specific, minimally invasive approach to managing these musculoskeletal complaints, utilising modalities such as ultrasound, CT, and fluoroscopy for both diagnosis and to guide treatment. Techniques including corticosteroid injections, dry needling, nerve hydrodissection, and orthobiologic therapies are tailored to specific pathologies, with the aim of providing symptomatic relief, whilst minimising the risk of complication, as well as time away from performance. Ultrasound is particularly valuable for due to its lack of ionising radiation, real-time capabilities, and exceptional soft tissue resolution. These interventions not provide pain relief, but also support musicians in maintaining performance and career longevity, underscoring the growing role of interventional radiology in occupational musculoskeletal care.

1 Introduction

Musculoskeletal (MSK) injuries in musicians generally relate to overuse syndromes, repetitive strain injuries or cumulative trauma, with manifestations including tendinopathy, tenosynovitis,

Med Radiol Diagn Imaging (2025)

https://doi.org/10.1007/174_2025_637,
Published Online: 12 November 2025

nerve entrapment, and osteoarthritis. The morbidity associated with these playing-related musculoskeletal disorders (PRMD) can impact performance and in cases of professional musicians, can have catastrophic consequences with regard to career progression (Rotter et al. 2019; Yang et al. 2021). Interventional radiology (IR) is the process by which procedures can be performed in a minimally invasive fashion, facilitated by the use of image guidance. This process can result in fewer complications than traditional surgical methods and in cases where accurate administration of a drug is necessary, radiological needle visualisation can optimise this, compared with anatomical landmark-based techniques (Arnold et al. 2019). The PRMD faced by musicians vary by instrument and are detailed elsewhere in this book. This chapter serves to describe the various imaging modalities and interventional techniques which can be utilised in the management of common disorders sustained by musicians.

2 Principles of Interventional Radiology in the Management of Musicians

The various procedures will be detailed in this section, following a discussion regarding the main imaging modalities used in MSK IR.

2.1 Imaging Modalities

Ultrasound is a low-cost, portable, non-ionising imaging modality, which provides excellent soft tissue resolution, particularly of superficial structures, such as tendons, muscles, and certain joints (Joines et al. 2007). Furthermore, it allows for dynamic assessment of structures, in contrast to static imaging modalities such as computed tomography (CT) and magnetic resonance imaging (MRI), which can increase its sensitivity for certain pathologies, such as tendon snapping and nerve subluxation. The dynamic capability of ultrasound also facilitates real-time needle visualisation during interventions which require precise needle positioning, either for dry needling or injection of medications, whilst ensuring to avoid adjacent soft tissue or neurovascular structures (Joines et al. 2007). In-plane and out-of-plane techniques can be utilised for ultrasound-guided procedures, with the needle appearing as a hyperechoic linear structure and a hyperechoic dot, respectively, in the two techniques (Joines et al. 2007). The specific ultrasound probe used varies depending on the anatomical location of the intervention being performed, with a higher frequency probe (e.g. 6–15 MHz) being used for more superficial procedures (e.g. hand and wrist) and a lower frequency probe (e.g. 1–6 MHz) used to visualise deeper structures (e.g. hip joint), owing to the improved ultrasound transmission at lower frequencies.

Fluoroscopically guided interventions in the MSK context really only comprise intra-articular injections and nerve root blocks. This is due to the modality's inability to accurately differentiate soft tissue structures, resulting in a reliance on osseous landmarks and tactile feedback from the needle during the procedure. Fluoroscopy is however exceedingly accurate with regard to intra-articular injections, with between 97% and 100% of injections being successful: a significantly greater proportion than landmark-guided injections (Saha et al. 2023). Appropriate positioning of the patient is key to both ensure optimal target visualisation, as well as to maximise patient comfort and safety. The X-ray tube should be positioned such that the injection target is located centrally in the image, and the entire joint is demonstrated (Kresse et al. 2023). Smaller joints are often more easily accessed by ultrasound, compared with fluoroscopy, and the need to confirm intra-articular needle position with contrast media in the latter modality can limit the volume of injectate the joint space can accommodate. This in turn can reduce the success of the procedure, given that a smaller volume of drug can be administered, potentially resulting in a shorter period of symptomatic relief for the patient.

Computed tomography (CT) has a limited role in the image-guided management of PRMD, with nerve root blocks forming the bulk of its utility. CT-guided interventions provide superior cross-sectional detail and spatial resolution, when compared with fluoroscopy, but come with an increased radiation dose to the patient (Dietrich et al. 2019). The dose to the operator however is reduced. The literature is variable regarding outcome measures of fluoroscopic versus CT, and more recently ultrasound-guided, nerve root block, with no clear consensus of which is superior (Dietrich et al. 2019; Kamp et al. 2022; Kimura et al. 2023).

2.2 Interventional Techniques

There are certain steps which are common to all MSK interventional procedures. First, the patient must be counselled regarding the intended benefits of the procedure, as well as the risks and potential complications. Once informed consent has been obtained, the patient must be appropriately positioned to optimise comfort for both the patient and practitioner, whilst also allowing the target site to be adequately imaged by the chosen modality, and sterile precautions must be utilised (Kresse et al. 2023; Rastogi et al. 2016).

Dry needling is a minimally invasive, cheap, and low risk interventional technique, which has emerged as a treatment option for patients suffering from myofascial pain: a common aetiology in musicians due to repetitive motions and often asymmetric posturing. Myofascial trigger points are identified either using landmark techniques or by ultrasound, as areas where a local muscle twitch response is elicited on palpation. These are thought to refer the pain that the patient experiences, secondary to motor dysfunction and autonomic nervous system dysregulation (Vas 2022). Placement of fine needles into these trigger points causes stimulation of the affected muscle or muscle groups, exhibited in the form of local twitches which eventually subside. This is believed to be due to the cessation of neural electrical activity, which reduces the abnormal motor stimulation. This, along with increasing blood flow to the area, is the theory behind improved patient symptoms (Kalichman and Vulfsons 2010). There is evidence of varying strengths that dry needling offers a benefit over no intervention or placebo in the management of myofascial pain. Dry needling has been shown to be equally as effective as multiple other MSK needling techniques for short- and medium-term symptomatic relief; however, local anaesthetic injections provide superior short-term relief (Chys et al. 2023). The benefits of using ultrasound in dry needling are multiple (Fig. 1). Low intensity muscle twitches are more sensitively identified by ultrasound, as well as trigger points in deeper muscles. Additionally, more accurate needle positioning can be achieved by using ultrasound, particularly in deeper muscles, and there is a lesser rate of complications relating to needle mispositioning, due to visualisation (Vas 2022).

Image-guided injections for MSK symptoms in musicians must utilise the correct drug to balance the speed of onset, intended duration of effect, safety profile, and potential tissue toxicity, given the urgent need to return to performance that professional musicians are often faced with. These injections can be performed in a range of locations for the treatment of pain, depending on the underlying aetiology, generally under either

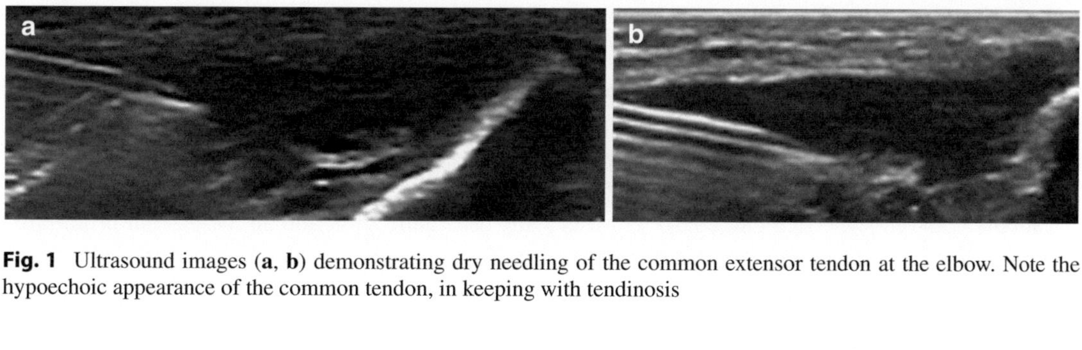

Fig. 1 Ultrasound images (**a**, **b**) demonstrating dry needling of the common extensor tendon at the elbow. Note the hypoechoic appearance of the common tendon, in keeping with tendinosis

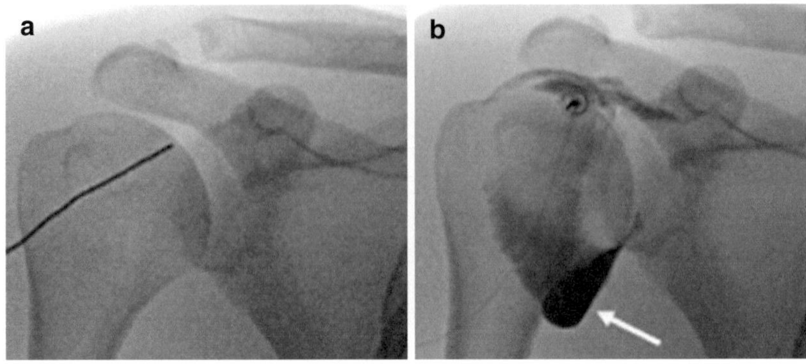

Fig. 2 Fluoroscopic hydrodilatation images demonstrating planning (**a**) and peri-injection (**b**). Note the radiopaque contrast media (arrow), which is used to confirm intra-articular needle position, prior to joint capsule distension

ultrasound or fluoroscopic guidance. Potential spaces for injection include into a joint, tendon sheath, muscle trigger point or bursa, as well as around tendons without sheaths or peripheral nerves (Patel et al. 2022; Rastogi et al. 2016).

Intra-articular injections can be performed under either fluoroscopic or sonographic guidance, depending on operator preference and departmental availability. Benefits of fluoroscopy include the ability to demonstrate definite intra-articular needle position, through contrast injection prior to instillation of the pharmaceutical, however unless an osseous backstop is used to determine the needle depth, the fluoroscopy tube must be angled orthogonally, to ensure an appropriate depth (Fig. 2). Ultrasound, on the other hand, allows for easier fine-tuning of needle trajectory and important soft tissue structures can be identified, such as neurovascular bundles, and therefore avoided (Rastogi et al. 2016). There is also the fact the ultrasound does not make use of ionising radiation, as fluoroscopy does (Figs. 3, 4, 5, 6, and 7).

Adhesive capsulitis is an insidious condition, most commonly affecting the glenohumeral joint (frozen shoulder), manifesting as capsular thickening, inflammation, and the formation of adhesions and scar tissue. Clinically, patients present with stiffness, reduced range of motion, pain, and dysfunction of the affected joint. Whilst literature relating adhesive capsulitis specifically to musicians is lacking, its incidence is approximately 3%–5% in the general population, rising to 20% in patients with diabetes (Le et al. 2016). For this reason, it is within the realms of possibility that some of the patients with this condition are musicians. *Hydrodilatation* is a recognised treatment strategy for this disorder, in which the joint is progressively injected with fluid, either up to a specified volume, often 30 mL or until capsular rupture is demonstrated by imaging. The fluid injected is commonly a combination of sterile saline and a local anaesthetic, with or without the addition of a corticosteroid. Recent meta-analysis has shown that hydrodilatation may provide benefit in the early stages of the disease with regard to disability and passive external rotation, but many of the long-term outcomes are comparable to intra-articular corticosteroid injection alone, without distension (Poku et al. 2023).

The instrument-specific pathologies are detailed elsewhere in this book; however, bursitis of varying locations is a common upper limb pathology which affects musicians who play instruments in the violin family. Affected sites in particular include the subacromial-subdeltoid and bicipitoradial bursae, due to repetitive shoulder abduction and elbow flexion, respectively (Schaefer and Speier 2012). The management of these conditions is generally conservative, with physiotherapy alone, or by supplementary corticosteroid *bursal injection*, to both reduce inflammation and provide a pain-free window in which to undertake physiotherapy (Fig. 8).

Tendon disease affecting musicians is typically mechanical in aetiology, secondary to the imbalance between repeated mechanical micro-injury and remodelling capability of the tendon. This process results in progressive collagen bundle disorganisation and an increase in proinflammatory cytokines, which stimulate intra- and peritendinous neovascularity, resulting in symp-

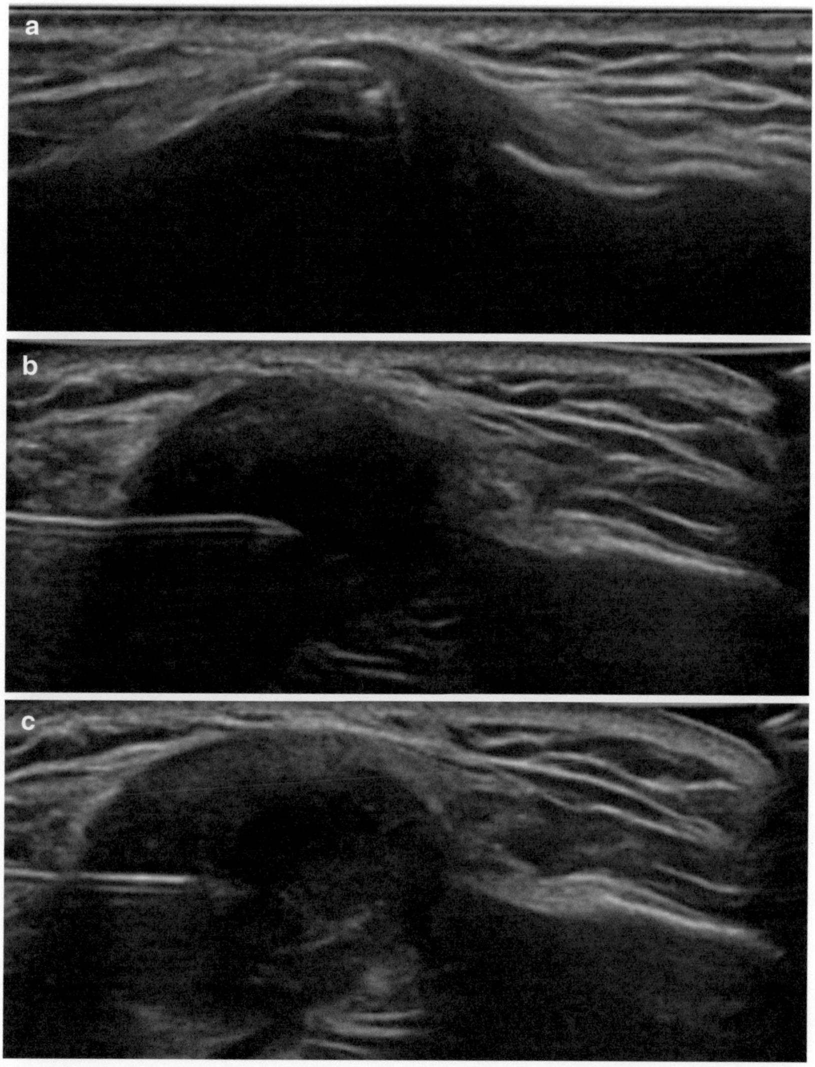

Fig. 3 Ultrasound image demonstrating a coronal oblique view of the acromioclavicular joint (**a**), followed by in-plane needle insertion (**b**) and intra-articular injection (**c**), with a perpendicular view

toms of pain, which can limit performance (Silva et al. 2023). *Image-guided tendon procedures* in the upper limb are typically performed under ultrasound guidance, with the aim of injecting a solution into a specific tendinous or peritendinous region, to either reduce the degree of inflammation or promote a healing response. These injections can be broadly divided in to peritendinous and intratendinous, with different injectates being used for each (Figs. 9 and 10). At the elbow, the distal biceps tendon is another structure which can generate pain in some musicians, secondary to repetitive elbow flexion and resultant tearing or tendinosis (Fig. 11). Ultrasound-guided injection of the tear or around the degenerate tendon with an orthobiologic substance, for example platelet-rich plasma, has yielded promising results, appearing to be effective and safe in small study cohorts. However, further investigations are required (Barker et al. 2015; Moreno-Garcia and Rodriguez-Merchan 2022). Musicians are at increased risk of De Quervain tenosynovitis with degeneration due to overuse from repetitive thumb and wrist movements, being an accepted mechanism. The combination of a corticosteroid injection into the tendon sheath of the first extensor compartment, followed by thumb spica immobilisation is widely accepted as the primary

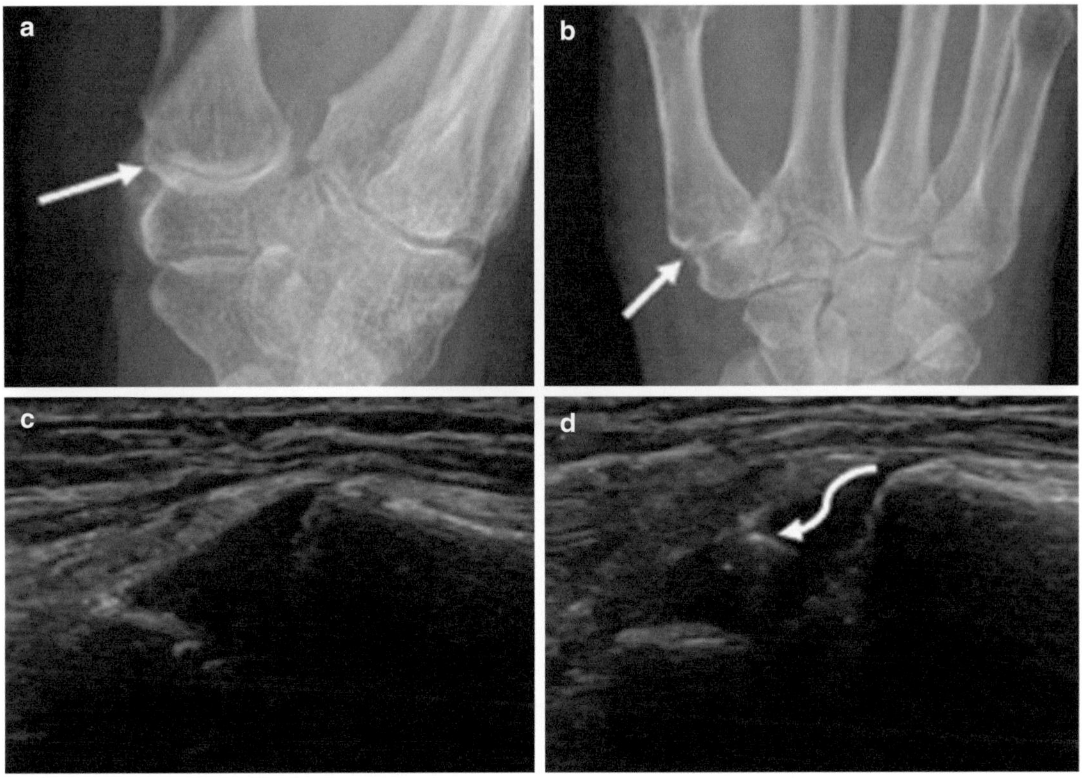

Fig. 4 Oblique radiographs (**a**, **b**) demonstrating osteoarthritis of the first carpometacarpal joint (straight arrows). Ultrasound image demonstrating the same joint (**c**), followed by an out-of-plane injection (**d**). Note the needle appearing as a hyperechoic dot (curved arrow)

treatment for this condition (Challoumas et al. 2023; Chong et al. 2024). The use of ultrasound guidance for needle positioning in this particular injection has not been shown to offer a benefit over an anatomical landmark-based approach, regarding pain relief or function (Fig. 12). However, ultrasound-guided injections demonstrated a lesser rate of corticosteroid related skin complications or De Quervain recurrence (Challoumas et al. 2023; Kuo et al. 2024).

Perineural injections can also be performed using sonographic, fluoroscopic, or CT guidance, depending on the location of the nerve implicated in the patient's presentation: either in the peripheries or spinal nerve roots. Peripheral nerve entrapment syndromes are common in musicians, particularly the median and ulnar nerves in the carpal and cubital tunnels, respectively, as well as thoracic outlet syndrome (Wilson et al. 2014). Both the radial and ulnar nerves can be demonstrated sonographically, displaying a honeycomb appearance in short axis and a corduroy appearance longitudinally, with expansion and hypoechoic changes seen in some cases of neuritis. Using in-plane ultrasound guidance, either perpendicular or parallel to the nerve, a 25G or 23G needle can be positioned adjacent to the epineurium and injectate infiltrated (Nwawka and Miller 2016). The needle generally needs to be slightly repositioned following the initial injection, in order to achieve circumferential coverage of the nerve with the injectate. For diagnostic injections, levobupivacaine 0.25% should be injected, due to its longer duration of action than lidocaine 1%, whilst in therapeutic injections, a corticosteroid can be added. The various injectates will be discussed subsequently within this chapter.

Nerve hydrodissection is the process by which a solution is injected around a peripheral nerve,

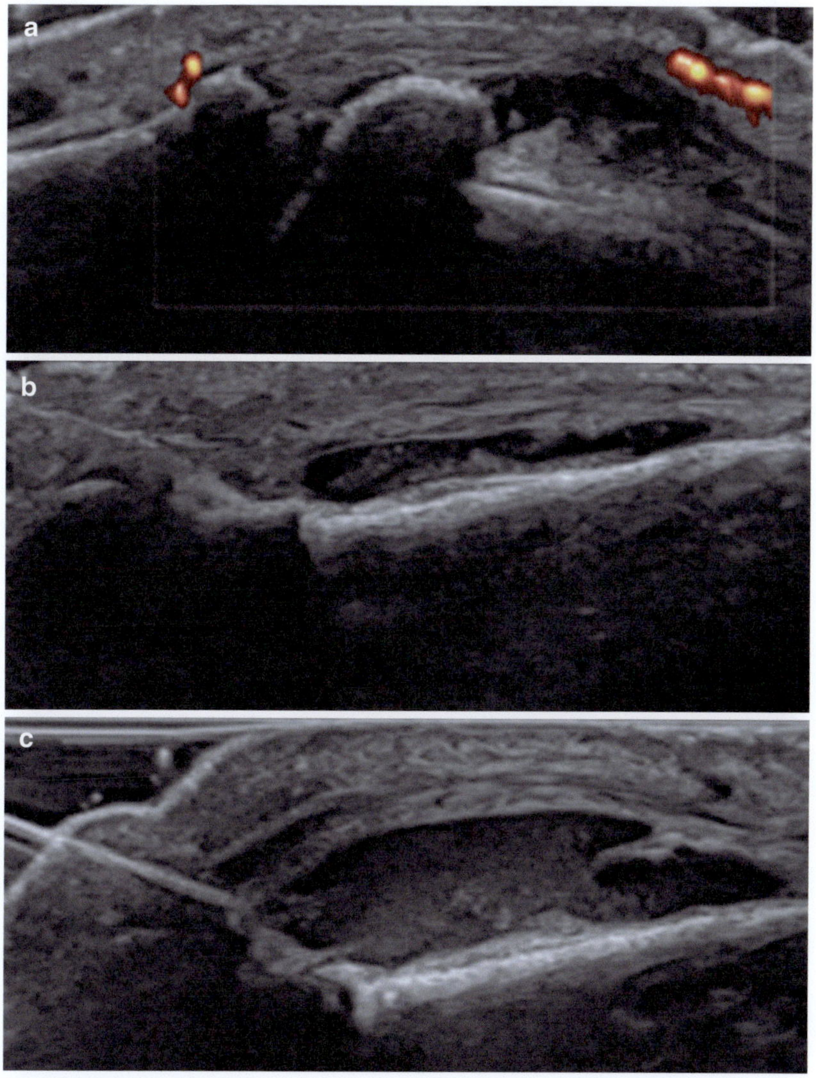

Fig. 5 Ultrasound images demonstrating a joint effusion and synovial proliferation in a proximal interphalangeal joint (**a**), followed by in-plane needle insertion (**b**) and injection (**c**)

specifically between the epineurium and more superficial adventitial glide layer, in order to both facilitate circumferential perineural medication spread, as well as to separate the nerve from the surrounding tissue, fascia, or adjacent structures (Fig. 13). It is hypothesised that adherence of the nerve to these structures contributes the nerve entrapment and therefore to the symptoms of the musician (Symanski et al. 2022). This procedure is performed under ultrasound guidance with direct in-plane visualisation of the needle, to minimise the risk of inadvertent neural injury (Lam et al. 2020). The median nerve in the carpal tunnel is a location which can be injected with either normal saline, local anaesthetic or dextrose in water, resulting in a therapeutic effect for patients with mild to moderate carpal tunnel syndrome. Additionally, this has been shown to be potentially beneficial to patients prior to surgery for carpal tunnel (Wu et al. 2019). This technique can be extrapolated to other sites of nerve entrapment, which affect musicians, such as the ulnar nerve in the cubital tunnel and in certain cases the sciatic and peroneal nerves in the gluteal and knee/ankle regions, respectively.

Radiculopathy, that is pain related to compression of a spinal nerve root, is common in the general population with annual prevalence of 486 and 83 per 100,000 per year, in the lumbar and cervical spine, respectively (Armon et al. 2025). Symptoms relating to nerve root compression in either of these locations can be exacerbated in musicians by virtue of the fixed, sometimes awkward, positioning required during playing (Schaefer and Speier 2012). In addition to conservative measures, such as physiotherapy, simple analgesia and making postural adjustments where possible, image-guided *nerve root injections* play a role in the rehabilitation and management of radicular symptoms. Originally performed using fluoroscopy, and more recently CT guidance, epidural steroid injections are commonly performed with the aim to both reduce the degree of pain experienced by the patient and to confirm the specific pain generator (Palmer 2016). In the cervical spine, injections are commonly performed with the patient supine and their head turned away from the side being targeted for injection. Following standard preparatory steps, a 22G or 21G needle is advanced to the posteroinferior aspect of the ipsilateral neural foramen, under fluoroscopic or CT guidance, close to the exiting nerve root and dorsal root ganglion. Following injection of a small volume of contrast media, to exclude intravascular needle positioning and display epiradicular spread, a mixture of local anaesthetic and non-particulate corticosteroid can be injected (Fig. 14). The importance of using non-particulate steroids is due to the potential for complication of cervical nerve root blocks, related to the abundant vasculature in the region of the dorsal root ganglion. Inadvertent injection of particulate steroid into the anterior radicular artery of the spinal cord, which is often not identified during image-guided intervention, can result in spinal cord infarction (Hodler et al. 2013). Moreover, an animal study demonstrated that particulate steroid injection into the vertebral artery caused brainstem and occipital infarction, resulting in the inability to self-ventilate and subsequent death (Hodler et al. 2013). There are a number of anatomical loca-

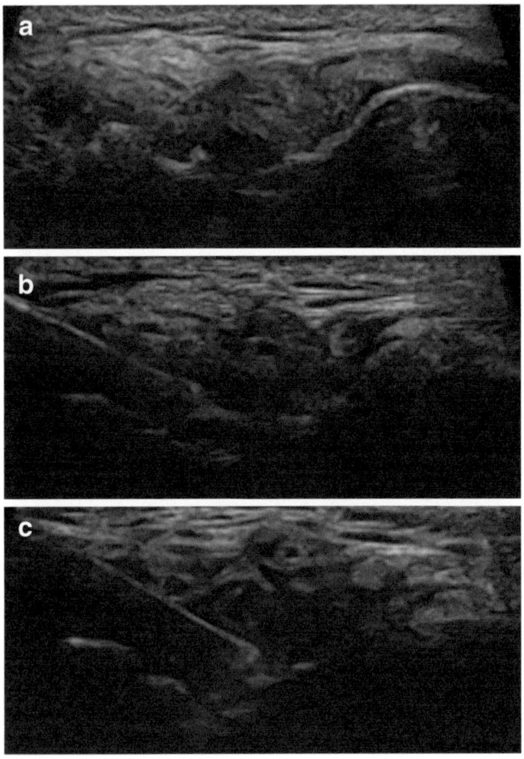

Fig. 6 Ultrasound images demonstrating a long axis view of the wrist joint at the level of the radiocarpal articulation (**a**), followed by in-plane needle insertion (**b**) and injection (**c**)

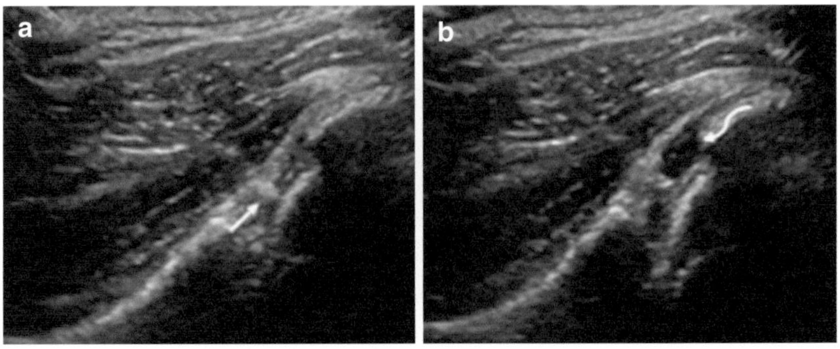

Fig. 7 Ultrasound images demonstrating a needle (arrow) positioned within the posterior aspect of the glenohumeral joint (**a**), followed by injection (**b**). Note the hypoechoic fluid, distending the posterior joint capsule (curved arrow)

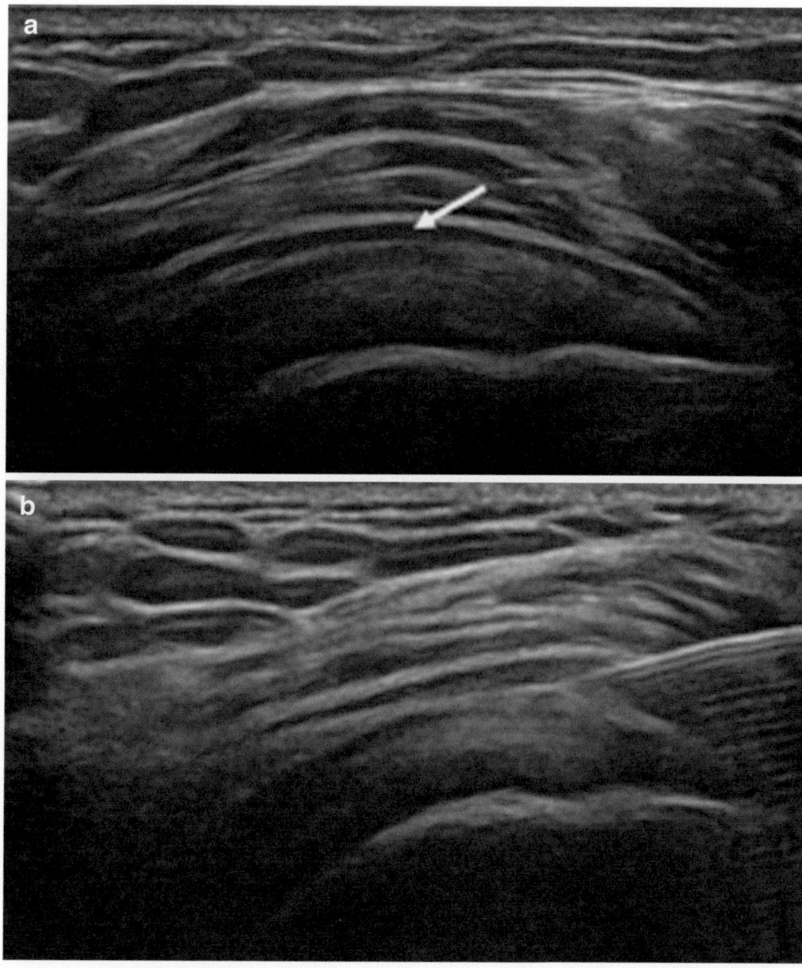

Fig. 8 Ultrasound image (**a**) demonstrating a small volume of hypoechoic fluid (arrow) in the subacromial-subdeltoid bursa, at the level of the supraspinatus tendon. This space was subsequently injected (**b**) with a mixture of local anaesthetic and steroid

tions which can be injected in the lumbar region, in addition the epidural space, including the facet joints, median branches, or synovial cysts, depending on the suspected site of pain generation (Palmer 2016). Lumbar epidural injections can also be performed fluoroscopically or under CT guidance. These injections are used to provide pain relief to patients suffering with 'sciatica', targeting the relevant lumbar nerve root (Fig. 15), and back pain, for which the affected facet joints is injected or relevant median branch blocked. Recently literature has been published suggesting similar efficacy of procedures performed under ultrasound guidance, compared with fluoroscopic guidance (Hofmeister et al. 2019; Wang et al. 2024). Whilst the use of ultrasound for these procedures comes with the obvious benefits of not using ionising radiation, not all patients will be appropriate candidates for this modality, depending on the target site for injection and patient habitus. Fluoroscopic or CT guidance remains advisable for epidural and transforaminal injections, given the inherent limitations of ultrasound when faced with cortical bone. The need for further studies assessing the utility of ultrasound in nerve root injections has been highlighted.

2.3 Injectates

Different *local anaesthetic* agents can be utilised for in these interventions, with specific medicines selected due to their onset, duration, and tissue

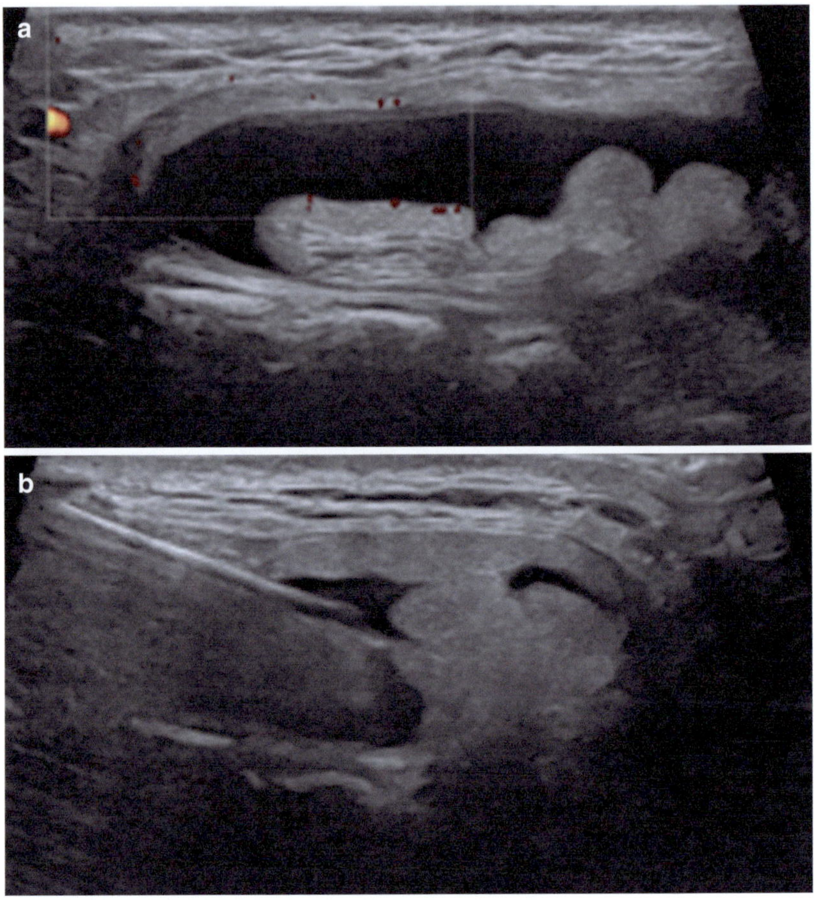

Fig. 9 Ultrasound image (**a**) demonstrating a large volume of hypoechoic fluid and synovial proliferation within the extensor digitorum communis tendon sheath at the wrist, in keeping with tenosynovitis. Using an in-plane approach (**b**), this fluid was aspirated and the tendon sheath subsequently injected

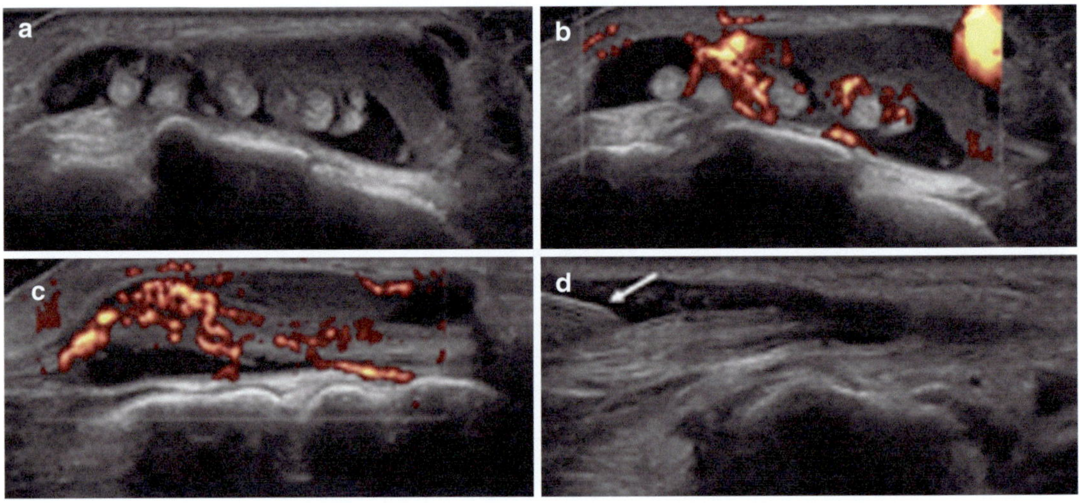

Fig. 10 Short axis (**a**, **b**) and long axis (**c**) ultrasound images demonstrating a moderate volume of hypoechoic fluid, synovial proliferation and increased vascularity within the 4th and 5th extensor compartments at the wrist, in keeping with tenosynovitis. Using an in-plane approach parallel to the tendons (**d**), the two compartments were sequentially injected (arrow showing needle tip)

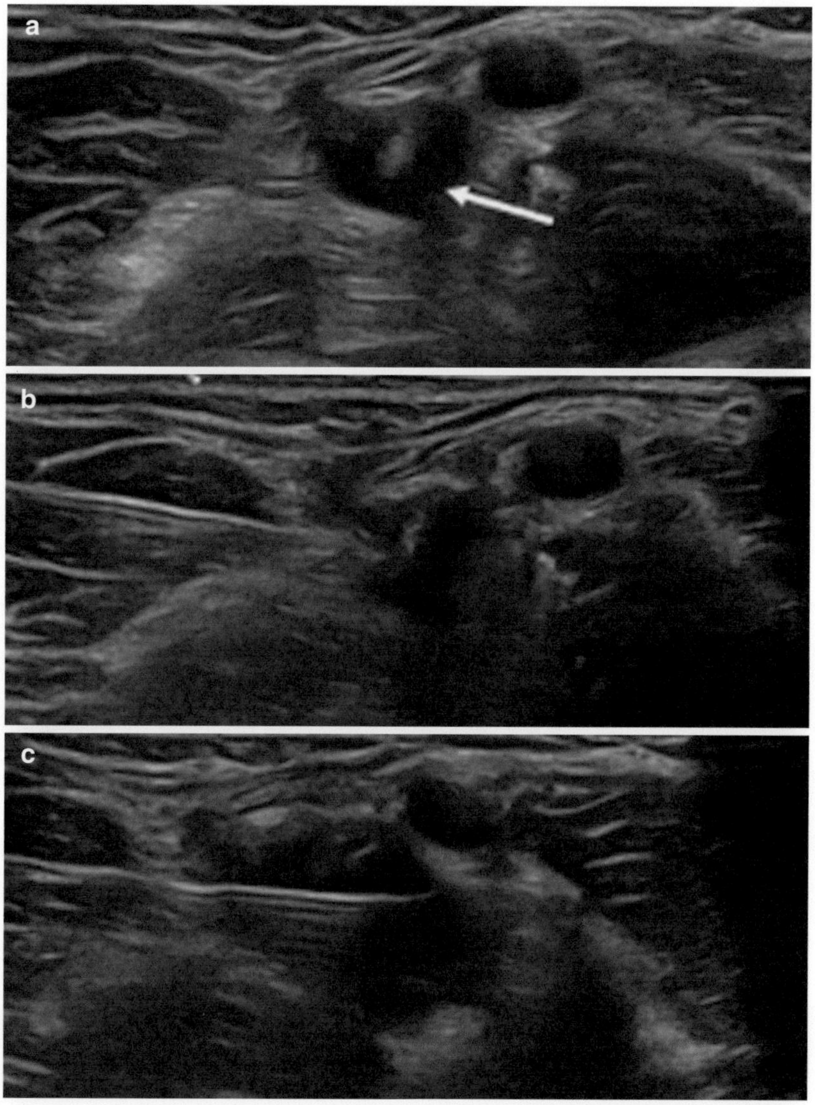

Fig. 11 Ultrasound image (**a**) demonstrates hypoechoic fluid (arrow) in the bicipitoradial bursa, surrounding the distal biceps tendon. Subsequent images demonstrate the insertion of a needle into this fluid (**b**), followed by injection (**c**)

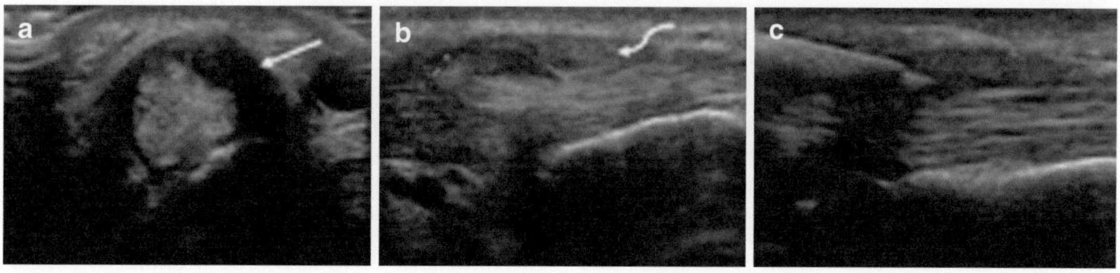

Fig. 12 Short axis (**a**) and long axis (**b**) ultrasound images demonstrating thickening of the extensor retinaculum (arrow) overlying the first extensor compartment tendons of the wrist, with synovial proliferation (curved arrow) within the tendon sheath. This space was injected via an in-plane approach (**c**)

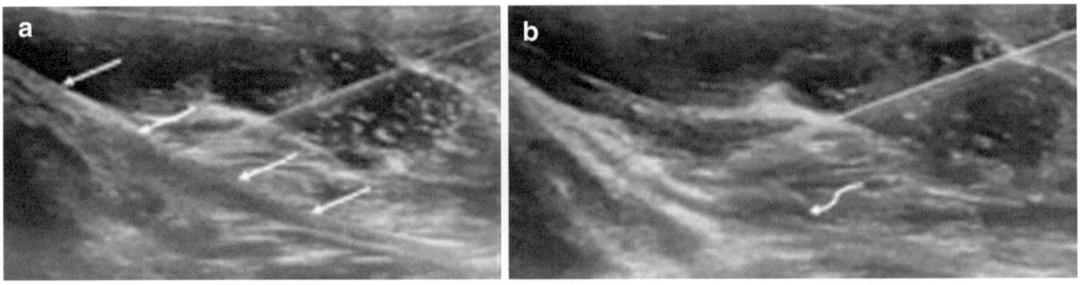

Fig. 13 Ultrasound image at the wrist (**a**) demonstrating a needle positioned adjacent to the epineurium of the median nerve (arrows). This space was subsequently injected (**b**) with a small volume of hypoechoic fluid (curved arrow) demonstrated to dissect between the nerve epineurium and the surrounding soft tissue

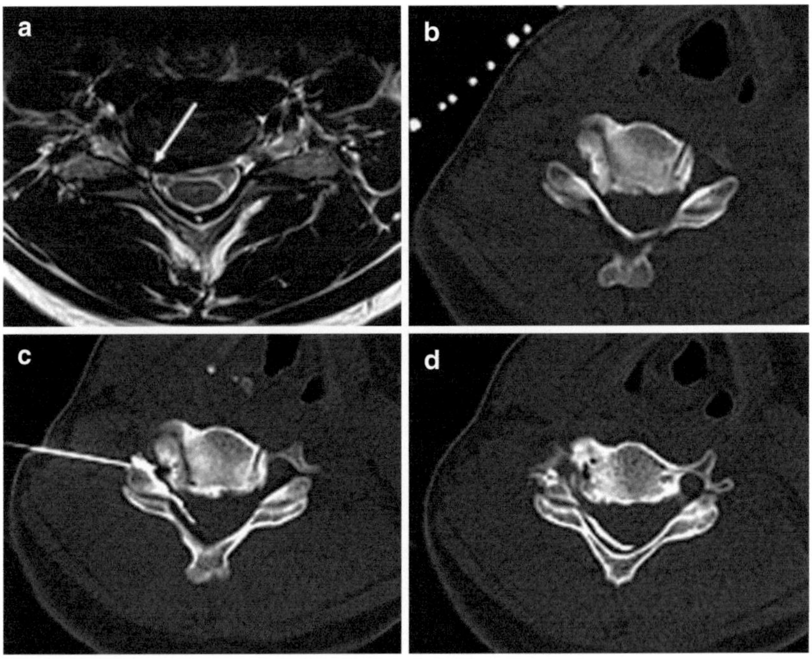

Fig. 14 MR (**a**) and CT (**b**) images demonstrating a right-sided disc-osteophyte complex (arrow) narrowing the right C5/6 neural foramen. Under CT guidance, a needle was positioned at the posterior aspect of the neural foramen and a small volume of iodinated contrast medium injected (**c**). Once intravascular needle positioning was excluded, the epidural space was subsequently injected (**d**). Note the posterior epidural spread of contrast

toxicity profiles. Amide anaesthetic agents are used in MSK injections, rather than esters, due to their lower risk of allergic reactions and more predictable metabolism. Lidocaine is the most commonly used, at least in the skin and soft tissues, due to its rapid onset, within 2 min, and intermediate duration, up to 2 h, providing near-immediate procedural pain relief. Bupivacaine and levobupivacaine, its less cardiotoxic S-enantiomer, have a longer duration of action, up to 6 h, however can take up to 10 min to act. Ropivacaine takes a similar length of time to act as bupivacaine, with effects lasting for 2–3 h (Caballero et al. 2022). The effect on tissues, specifically chondrocytes and tenocytes, is another factor which must be considered when selecting the anaesthetic to be injected. Ropivacaine has been demonstrated as the least chondrotoxic of the three aforementioned drugs, and is also the least cardiotoxic, in case of inadvertent intravascular injection. Lidocaine is the least toxic to the central nervous system; however, it is relatively chondrotoxic, making it a poor choice for intra-articular injection.

Corticosteroids are injected due to their anti-inflammatory effects, making them beneficial in the treatment of bursitis and tenosynovitis. Triamcinolone acetonide and methylpredniso-

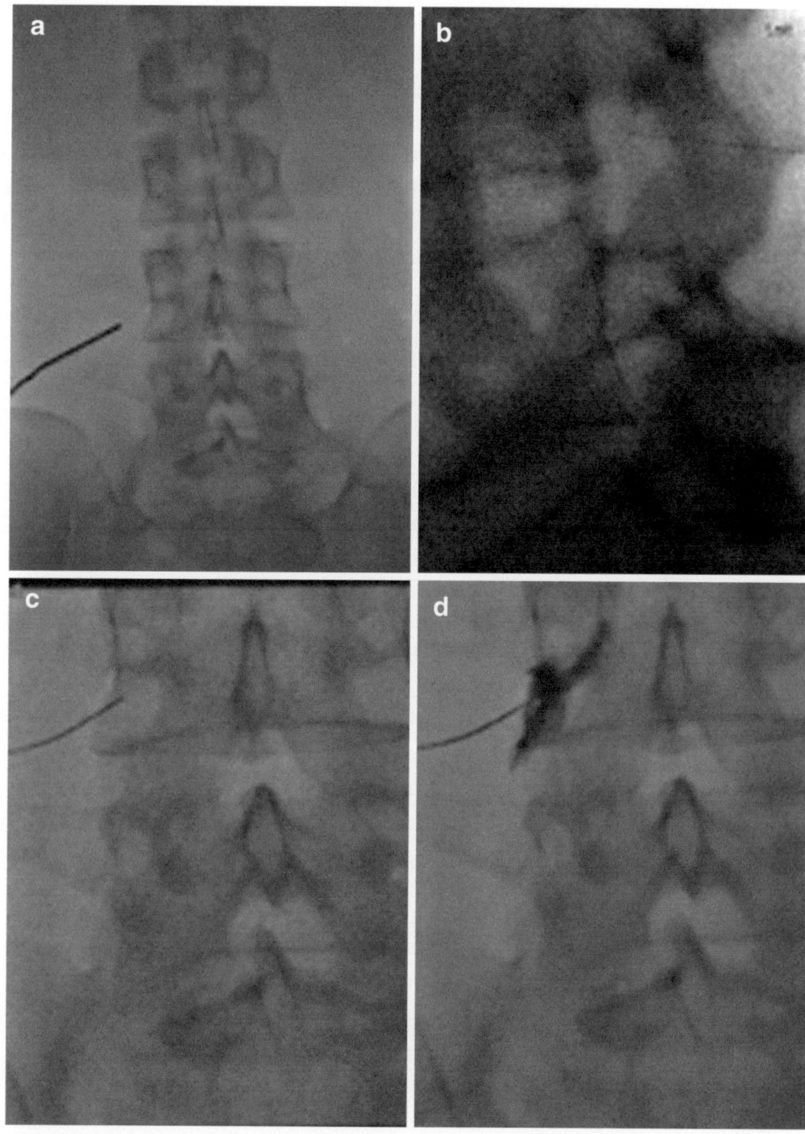

Fig. 15 Planning PA fluoroscopic image (**a**) demonstrating a radiopaque marker, positioned in the region of the left L4/5 neural foramen (note the patient's prone position). Subsequent lateral (**b**) and PA (**c**) fluoroscopy images demonstrate needle positioning in the safe triangle, followed by confirmation of positioning with iodinated contrast medium and subsequent injection (**d**)

lone acetate are particulate corticosteroid suspensions, commonly injected in the MSK intervention setting. It is important to restrict these to bursae and tendon sheaths, due to their potential for causing tendon damage or rupture, if injected into the tendon substance (Silva et al. 2023). No clinically significant difference in efficacy has been demonstrated between the two drugs, and triamcinolone acetonide is considered to have a slightly longer duration of action, due to its lower solubility and slower absorption (Shahinfar and Maibach 2023). In the context of nerve root injections, it is imperative to use a soluble corticosteroid, such as dexamethasone, rather than a particulate suspension. This relates to the potential for corticosteroid particles to form aggregates and embolise into the arterioles of the spine and brain, resulting in infarction, in addition to the catastrophic consequences of unintended arterial injection demonstrated in animal studies (Hodler et al. 2013; Munglani et al. 2020).

Orthobiologic is an umbrella term encompassing a range of therapies, which include blood- and tissue-based substances. An exhaustive description of all of the current orthobiologics is beyond the scope of this chapter, given the ever-increasing number of available therapies and their clinical applications. Instead, some of the more established agents will be summarised. *Platelet-rich plasma* (PRP) is derived from centrifuged autologous blood, resulting in an injectate that has a platelet concentration between 3 and 8 times more than is found in whole blood—defined as at least 1,000,000 platelets/mL (Su et al. 2022). The ideal concentration of platelets within this range is yet to be defined, but evidence suggests between 2.5 and 6 times greater than that of whole blood is optimal, with greater concentrations potentially slowing the healing process. Subdivisions of PRP include leukocyte-rich and leukocyte-poor PRP, referring to the leukocyte concentration, relative to the standard. The current applications for PRP are vast, including shoulder intra-articular injection for adhesive capsulitis, peritendinous injection for tendinopathy and tenosynovitis, particularly at the first extensor compartment of the wrist in De Quervain disease (Rosso et al. 2023; Silva et al. 2023). *Autologous whole blood* is a less processed injectate than PRP, with both hypothesised to induce healing at sites of degeneration, by providing cellular and humoral mediators (Rabago et al. 2008). The injection of *hyaluronic acid* (HA), an important component in articular cartilage and synovial fluid, has been reported as a beneficial orthobiologic for osteoarthritis of large joints. There is limited clinical data available regarding HA use in tendinopathies; a pathology more relevant to musicians, and whilst HA is reported as safe and modestly effective, the evidence supports PRP as providing greater and more durable clinical benefit, in most comparative studies (Kubrova et al. 2020). *Prolotherapy* is the injection of an irritant solution, most commonly hyperosmolar dextrose, which is postulated to encourage healing of damaged musculoskeletal soft tissue structures, including tendons, ligaments, fascial structures, and cartilage (Rabago and Nourani 2017). Such conditions where prolotherapy efficacy has been demonstrated include lateral epicondylitis and rotator cuff degeneration (Bertrand et al. 2016; Rabago et al. 2013; Scarpone et al. 2008).

3 Conclusion

The role of IR in the management of PRMD in musicians requires an understanding of the unique biomechanical demands placed on this population and a nuanced understanding of the various tools available. Through IR, precise, minimally invasive procedures can be performed to target specific anatomical sites, to improve symptoms, while minimising recovery time: a key consideration for musicians under pressure to maintain performance standards. Ultrasound is the modality most frequently utilised modality for intervention, owing to its dynamic capabilities and lack of radiation; however, fluoroscopy and CT are currently indispensable for nerve root injections. The wide range of interventions from dry needling to orthobiologic injection can be tailored to specific PRMD. The efficacy and potential tissue toxicity of the injectate must be considered, depending on whether the injection is peritendinous, intratendinous, or intra-articular, and both hydrodissection and perineural injections offer therapeutic avenues for entrapment syndromes, common among musicians. To summarise, the role of IR for musicians is significant, facilitating personalised, safe, and effective treatment strategies to not only alleviate symptoms, but also support long-term functional recovery.

References

Armon C, Narayanaswami P, Potrebic S, Gronseth G, Bačkonja MM, Cai VL, Dorman J, Gilligan C, Heller SA, Silsbee HM, Smith DB (2025) Epidural steroids for cervical and lumbar radicular pain and spinal stenosis systematic review summary: report of the AAN Guidelines Subcommittee. Neurology 104:e213361. https://doi.org/10.1212/WNL.0000000000213361/SUPPL_FILE/EAPPENDIX_1.PDF

Arnold MJ, Keung JJ, McCarragher B (2019) Interventional radiology: indications and best practices. Am Fam Physician 99:547–556

Barker SL, Bell SN, Connell D, Coghlan JA (2015) Ultrasound-guided platelet-rich plasma injection for distal biceps tendinopathy. Shoulder Elbow 7:110. https://doi.org/10.1177/1758573214567558

Bertrand H, Reeves KD, Bennett CJ, Bicknell S, Cheng AL (2016) Dextrose prolotherapy versus control injections in painful rotator cuff tendinopathy. Arch Phys

Med Rehabil 97:17–25. https://doi.org/10.1016/j.apmr.2015.08.412

Caballero M, Kobayashi Y, Gottschalk AW (2022) Local anesthetic use in musculoskeletal injections. Ochsner J 22:200. https://doi.org/10.31486/TOJ.22.0061

Challoumas D, Ramasubbu R, Rooney E, Seymour-Jackson E, Putti A, Millar NL (2023) Management of de Quervain tenosynovitis: a systematic review and network meta-analysis. JAMA Netw Open 6:e2337001. https://doi.org/10.1001/JAMANETWORKOPEN.2023.37001

Chong HH, Pradhan A, Dhingra M, Liong W, Hau MYT, Shah R (2024) Advancements in de Quervain tenosynovitis management: a comprehensive network meta-analysis. J Hand Surg 49:557–569. https://doi.org/10.1016/j.jhsa.2024.03.003

Chys M, De Meulemeester K, De Greef I, Murillo C, Kindt W, Kouzouz Y, Lescroart B, Cagnie B (2023) Clinical effectiveness of dry needling in patients with musculoskeletal pain—an umbrella review. J Clin Med 12:1205. https://doi.org/10.3390/JCM12031205/S1

Dietrich TJ, Peterson CK, Zeimpekis KG, Bensler S, Sutter R, Pfirrmann CWA (2019) Fluoroscopy-guided versus CT-guided lumbar steroid injections: comparison of radiation exposure and outcomes. Radiology 290:752–759. https://doi.org/10.1148/RADIOL.2018181224/ASSET/IMAGES/LARGE/RADIOL.2018181224.TBL2.JPEG

Hodler J, Boos N, Schubert M (2013) Must we discontinue selective cervical nerve root blocks?: Report of two cases and review of the literature. Eur Spine J 22:466. https://doi.org/10.1007/S00586-012-2642-Z

Hofmeister M, Dowsett LE, Lorenzetti DL, Clement F (2019) Ultrasound- versus fluoroscopy-guided injections in the lower back for the management of pain: a systematic review. Eur Radiol 29:3401–3409. https://doi.org/10.1007/S00330-019-06065-3/TABLES/2

Joines MM, Motamedi K, Seeger LL, DiFiori JP (2007) Musculoskeletal interventional ultrasound. Semin Musculoskelet Radiol 11:192–198. https://doi.org/10.1055/S-2007-1001883

Kalichman L, Vulfsons S (2010) Dry needling in the management of musculoskeletal pain. J Am Board Fam Med 23:640–646. https://doi.org/10.3122/JABFM.2010.05.090296

Kamp JPM, Bartlett J, Fahmy A, To K, Hossain R, Akula M (2022) CT-guided vs. fluoroscopically guided transforaminal epidural steroid injections for lumbar radiculopathy: a comparison of efficacy, safety and cost. Arch Orthop Trauma Surg 143:2355. https://doi.org/10.1007/S00402-022-04436-Y

Kimura R, Yamamoto N, Watanabe J, Ono Y, Hongo M, Miyakoshi N (2023) Comparative efficacy of ultrasound guidance and fluoroscopy or computed tomography guidance in spinal nerve injections: a systematic review and meta-analysis. Eur Spine J 32:4101–4110. https://doi.org/10.1007/S00586-023-07968-Y/FIGURES/5

Kresse ME, Perry MT, Nacey NC (2023) Fluoroscopy-guided injections of the upper extremity: pearls and pitfalls. Skeletal Radiol 52:843–854. https://doi.org/10.1007/S00256-022-04129-Y/FIGURES/15

Kubrova E, D'Souza RS, Hunt CL, Wang Q, Van Wijnen AJ, Qu W (2020) Injectable biologics: what is the evidence? Am J Phys Med Rehabil 99:950–960. https://doi.org/10.1097/PHM.0000000000001407

Kuo YC, Hsieh LF, Liu YF, Chang CS (2024) Ultrasound versus palpation-guided corticosteroid injection for de Quervain disease: a randomized controlled trial. PM R 16:948–958. https://doi.org/10.1002/PMRJ.13144

Lam KHS, Hung CY, Chiang YP, Onishi K, Su DCJ, Clark TB, Reeves KD (2020) Ultrasound-guided nerve hydrodissection for pain management: rationale, methods, current literature, and theoretical mechanisms. J Pain Res 13:1957. https://doi.org/10.2147/JPR.S247208

Le HV, Lee SJ, Nazarian A, Rodriguez EK (2016) Adhesive capsulitis of the shoulder: review of pathophysiology and current clinical treatments. Shoulder Elbow 9:75. https://doi.org/10.1177/1758573216676786

Moreno-Garcia A, Rodriguez-Merchan EC (2022) Orthobiologics: current role in orthopedic surgery and traumatology. Arch Bone Jt Surg 10:536. https://doi.org/10.22038/ABJS.2021.52770.2614

Munglani R, Knaggs R, Eyre G (2020) Particulate steroids in axial spinal blockade and the increasing role of patient consent: Les grains de sable dans l'engrenage. Br J Pain 14:141. https://doi.org/10.1177/2049463720921199

Nwawka OK, Miller TT (2016) Ultrasound-guided peripheral nerve injection techniques. Am J Roentgenol 207:507–516. https://doi.org/10.2214/AJR.16.16378/ASSET/IMAGES/LARGE/09_16_16378_10B.JPEG

Palmer WE (2016) Spinal injections for pain management. Radiology 281:669–688. https://doi.org/10.1148/RADIOL.2016152055/ASSET/IMAGES/LARGE/RADIOL.2016152055.FIG16B.JPEG

Patel RP, McGill K, Motamedi D, Morgan T (2022) Ultrasound-guided interventions of the upper extremity joints. Skeletal Radiol 52:897. https://doi.org/10.1007/S00256-022-04148-9

Poku D, Hassan R, Migliorini F, Maffulli N (2023) Efficacy of hydrodilatation in frozen shoulder: a systematic review and meta-analysis. Br Med Bull 147:121. https://doi.org/10.1093/BMB/LDAD018

Rabago D, Nourani B (2017) Prolotherapy for osteoarthritis and tendinopathy: a descriptive review. Curr Rheumatol Rep 19:1–8. https://doi.org/10.1007/S11926-017-0659-3/TABLES/1

Rabago D, Best TM, Zgierska AE, Zeisig E, Ryan M, Crane D (2008) A systematic review of four injection therapies for lateral epicondylosis: prolotherapy, polidocanol, whole blood and platelet rich plasma. Br J Sports Med 43:471. https://doi.org/10.1136/BJSM.2008.052761

Rabago D, Lee KS, Ryan M, Chourasia AO, Sesto ME, Zgierska A, Kijowski R, Grettie J, Wilson J, Miller D (2013) Hypertonic dextrose and morrhuate sodium injections (prolotherapy) for lateral epicondylosis (tennis elbow): results of a single-blind, pilot-level, randomized controlled trial. Am J Phys Med Rehabil 92:587–596. https://doi.org/10.1097/PHM.0B013E31827D695F

Rastogi AK, Davis KW, Ross A, Rosas HG (2016) Fundamentals of joint injection. Am J Roentgenol 207:484–494. https://doi.org/10.2214/AJR.16.16243/ASSET/IMAGES/LARGE/09_16_16243_07E.JPEG

Rosso C, Morrey ME, Schär MO, Grezda K (2023) The role of platelet-rich plasma in shoulder pathologies: a critical review of the literature. EFORT Open Rev 8:213. https://doi.org/10.1530/EOR-22-0104

Rotter G, Noeres K, Fernholz I, Willich SN, Schmidt A, Berghöfer A (2019) Musculoskeletal disorders and complaints in professional musicians: a systematic review of prevalence, risk factors, and clinical treatment effects. Int Arch Occup Environ Health 93:149. https://doi.org/10.1007/S00420-019-01467-8

Saha P, Smith M, Hasan K (2023) Accuracy of intraarticular injections: blind vs. image guided techniques—a review of literature. J Funct Morphol Kinesiol 8:93. https://doi.org/10.3390/JFMK8030093

Scarpone M, Rabago DP, Zgierska A, Arbogast G, Snell E (2008) The efficacy of prolotherapy for lateral epicondylosis: a pilot study. Clin J Sport Med 18:248–254. https://doi.org/10.1097/JSM.0B013E318170FC87

Schaefer PT, Speier J (2012) Common medical problems of instrumental athletes. Curr Sports Med Rep 11:316–322. https://doi.org/10.1249/JSR.0B013E318272C8AE

Shahinfar S, Maibach H (2023) Enigma of intramuscular triamcinolone acetonide (Kenalog®) efficacy. Clin Pharmacokinet 62:1189–1199. https://doi.org/10.1007/S40262-023-01297-5/FIGURES/8

Silva FD, Zorzenoni F, da Silva LNM, dos Reis Teixeira Neto A, Gonzalez MT, Filho AGO, Guimarães JB (2023) Tendon injections – upper extremity. Skeletal Radiol 52:979–990. https://doi.org/10.1007/S00256-022-04174-7/FIGURES/5

Su CA, Jildeh TR, Vopat ML, Waltz RA, Millett PJ, Provencher MT, Philippon MJ, Huard J (2022) Current state of platelet-rich plasma and cell-based therapies for the treatment of osteoarthritis and tendon and ligament injuries. J Bone Joint Surg 104:1406–1414. https://doi.org/10.2106/JBJS.21.01112

Symanski JS, Ross AB, Davis KW, Brunner MC, Lee KS (2022) US for traumatic nerve injury, entrapment neuropathy, and imaging-guided perineural injection. Radiographics 42:1546–1561. https://doi.org/10.1148/RG.210152/RG210152SUPPM3.MP4

Vas LC (2022) Ultrasound guided dry needling: relevance in chronic pain. J Postgrad Med 68:1. https://doi.org/10.4103/JPGM.JPGM_710_21

Wang B, Sun Y, Zhang J, Meng H, Zhang H, Shan L (2024) Ultrasound-guided versus fluoroscopy-guided lumbar selective nerve root block: a retrospective comparative study. Sci Rep 14:3235. https://doi.org/10.1038/S41598-024-53809-3

Wilson RJ, Watson JT, Lee DH (2014) Nerve entrapment syndromes in musicians. Clin Anat 27:861–865. https://doi.org/10.1002/CA.22377

Wu YT, Chen SR, Li TY, Ho TY, Shen YP, Tsai CK, Chen LC (2019) Nerve hydrodissection for carpal tunnel syndrome: a prospective, randomized, double-blind, controlled trial. Muscle Nerve 59:174–180. https://doi.org/10.1002/MUS.26358

Yang N, Fufa DT, Wolff AL (2021) A musician-centered approach to management of performance-related upper musculoskeletal injuries. J Hand Ther 34:208–216. https://doi.org/10.1016/j.jht.2021.04.006

Correction to: Injuries Specific to Vocal Music and Radiological Features

Suhel Hasan, Smita Caren Mathias, Muralidhar K., and Kanaka Durga Prasad Bhamidipaty

Correction to:
Chapter 631 in: K. D. P. Bhamidipaty (ed.) et al., Med Radiol Diagn Imaging (2025), https://doi.org/10.1007/174_2025_631

The original version of this chapter was inadvertently published with the omission of the co-authors Suhel Hasan and Smita Caren Mathias, which has now been corrected. The author byline should read: Suhel Hasan, Smita Caren Mathias, Muralidhar K., and Kanaka Durga Prasad Bhamidipaty

The updated version of this chapter can be found at
https://doi.org/10.1007/174_2025_631

Med Radiol Diagn Imaging (2026)
https://doi.org/10.1007/978-3-032-14365-5_658,

MIX
Papier aus verantwortungsvollen Quellen
Paper from responsible sources
FSC® C105338

If you have any concerns about our products,
you can contact us on
ProductSafety@springernature.com

In case Publisher is established outside the EU,
the EU authorized representative is:
Springer Nature Customer Service Center GmbH
Europaplatz 3, 69115 Heidelberg, Germany

Printed by Libri Plureos GmbH
in Hamburg, Germany